ELYSANDRA EIRENE CALLISTA

Her Fast, Her Freedom - Innovavista Publishing

Contents

1

Introduction: The Tapestry of Timeless Wisdom

In a world brimming with information, where every scroll and click brings a barrage of knowledge, it's easy to be overwhelmed. The multitude of voices, each vying for attention, creates a cacophony that can drown out the whisper of intuition and the gentle guidance of personal experience. Amidst this noise, "Her Fast, Her Freedom" is not just a book but a sanctuary—a realm where wisdom meets wonder, science entwines with stories, and the modern woman discovers her ancient soul.

This book's architecture is unique. Imagine walking into a grand library, where each chamber holds its treasures, tales, and teachings. These chambers, akin to the chapters in this book, are standalone realms. Each is a microcosm, a complete universe of knowledge, waiting to be explored and experienced. You can wander into any chamber, at any moment, and immerse yourself without needing to trace back to another room or anticipate the next. Yet, for those who embark on the journey from the very first chamber to the last, an intricate tapestry of interwoven threads reveals itself—a symphony of harmonious melodies that resounds with the timeless rhythms of womanhood.

Now, let's embark on a brief journey through the hallways of time to understand the genesis of this tapestry.

Centuries ago, in an ancient civilization, the women were known as the "Guardians of Seasons." They weren't just keepers of time but the custodians of life's rhythms. They understood that the world around them—the waxing and waning of the moon, the flow of rivers, the blossoming of flowers— all echoed the cycles within them. These women had a profound, sacred knowledge: the art of fasting. This was not a mere act of abstention but a deep, spiritual communion—a dance with the very essence of life.

As generations passed, this art was handed down, but not merely as ritualistic traditions. With each passing, it evolved, amalgamating with the wisdom of the age, incorporating the discoveries of science, the experiences of women, and the teachings of sages. This vast, boundless knowledge, however, faced the threats of time. Wars, migrations, and the sands of time threatened to disperse and dissolve this wisdom.

In one such era, a visionary named Lysandra, aware of the impending loss, embarked on a quest. Traveling through diverse lands, she met wise women from every corner of the world. From them, she gathered stories, experiences, methods, and insights. And she began penning down what would one day become "Her Fast, Her Freedom." Lysandra envisioned a book that would serve as a beacon—a lighthouse in the stormy seas of time, ensuring that the wisdom of the "Guardians of Seasons" was never lost.

Today, as you hold this book, know that it is not merely a compilation of words and wisdom. It is the legacy of countless women, the dreams of visionaries like Lysandra, and the collective consciousness of the "Guardians of Seasons." It is a bridge that spans across time, connecting ancient rituals with modern science, ancestral memory with contemporary experience.

Every chapter you delve into is both a portal and a sanctuary. Whether you're seeking guidance on hormonal harmony, understanding the nuances of female metabolism, or exploring the connection between fasting and mental well-being, each chapter offers a treasure trove of insights. They stand firm on their own, like majestic pillars, yet, when viewed from a distance, they form a grand edifice—a testament to the eternal and evolving journey of feminine fasting.

As you navigate these pages, remember Lysandra's vision—a book that serves, not as a prescriptive doctrine, but as a compass, always pointing you back to your essence, your intuition, your power. Here, you'll find scientific facts entwined with personal stories, ancient rituals juxtaposed against modern-day practices. The dualities merge to create a holistic, comprehensive guide—one that respects the unique journey of every woman while celebrating the collective wisdom of womankind.

Embark on this journey not just as a reader but as a seeker—a guardian of your seasons, a custodian of your rhythms, and a dancer in the eternal ballet of life. Whether you choose to wander through these chambers in order or let intuition guide your path, know that you're retracing the steps of countless women before you. And in doing so, you're not just learning but also contributing to the legacy, enriching the tapestry, and ensuring that "Her Fast, Her Freedom" remains a beacon for generations to come.

In the end, this isn't just a book; it's a universe, a legacy, a dance. Welcome to the timeless journey of "Her Fast, Her Freedom." Let the exploration begin.

2

The Science of Fasting and Fat Loss

Understanding the Metabolic Shift: From Glucose Burning to Fat Burning

Our bodies are incredible machines. They can adapt and switch between different energy sources depending on what's available. One of the most crucial shifts that can occur within our metabolism is moving from burning glucose (sugar) to burning fat. This transition isn't just about weight loss it's about optimizing our health, energy, and longevity.

When we eat a meal, especially one rich in carbohydrates, our body breaks down those carbohydrates into glucose. This glucose then enters our bloodstream, and our blood sugar levels rise. To manage this rise in blood sugar, our pancreas releases insulin, a hormone that helps cells take in glucose for energy or storage. When our cells have enough energy, any excess glucose gets stored as glycogen in the liver and muscles or as fat in fat cells.

This storage system is a survival mechanism. In the past, food wasn't always readily available. Storing excess energy as fat ensured that we had reserves to tap into during times of scarcity. However, in today's world, where food is abundant and often consumed in excess, this ancient system can work against us, leading to weight gain and related health issues.

For most people, the primary source of energy is glucose. It's quick, efficient, and readily available, especially if the diet is rich in carbohydrates. However, when we fast or substantially reduce our carbohydrate intake, something fascinating happens. Our glucose reserves start to deplete, especially the glycogen stored in the liver. When these reserves get low, the body begins to look for an alternative energy source: fat.

This switch to burning fat for fuel is called ketosis. When our body breaks down fats, it produces molecules called ketones. These ketones, especially beta-hydroxybutyrate (BHB), become the primary energy source for many cells, including brain cells. This switch has numerous benefits, from weight loss to enhanced mental clarity and reduced inflammation.

But how does fasting play into this? Fasting is one of the most effective ways to induce this metabolic shift. When we refrain from eating, our glucose levels drop, insulin levels decrease, and the body starts to burn stored fat for energy. This is the body's natural response to periods of food scarcity, ensuring that we can still function and thrive even when food is not available.

However, the benefits of this metabolic shift aren't limited to just weight loss. Burning fat for fuel, particularly in the form of ketones, has been shown to have several health benefits:

Brain Health: Ketones are a highly efficient fuel for the brain. They can enhance cognitive function, improve memory, and even have potential therapeutic effects for neurological disorders like epilepsy and Alzheimer's disease.

Reduced Inflammation: Ketosis has been shown to reduce markers of inflammation in the body, which can contribute to chronic diseases and aging.

Hormonal Balance: Fasting and ketosis can help regulate hormones related to hunger, stress, and growth. This can lead to improved mood, better sleep, and enhanced muscle preservation and growth.

Autophagy: This is a cellular "clean-up" process that gets activated during fasting. It helps remove damaged cells and cellular components, leading to rejuvenation and potential anti-aging effects.

Understanding this metabolic shift is essential for anyone looking to harness the power of fasting or a low-carbohydrate diet for weight loss and health optimization. It's not just about eating less or cutting out certain foods. It's about tapping into our body's innate ability to switch energy sources, adapt, and thrive.

While the journey from glucose burning to fat burning might seem daunting at first, with the right knowledge and tools, anyone can achieve it. As we delve deeper into this chapter, we'll explore the intricacies of this transition, the physiological processes involved, and how to optimize this shift for maximum health benefits.

In the subsequent sections, we'll also discuss common misconceptions about fasting, delve into the science of fat loss, and provide actionable steps to harness the power of this ancient practice in today's modern world. Remember, our bodies are adaptable machines. By understanding and working with our metabolism, we can unlock a world of potential for health, longevity, and vitality.

Exploring the Female Metabolism: A Unique Entity

When it comes to the world of metabolism, one size does not fit all. The female metabolism is a unique and intricate system that operates differently than its male counterpart. This distinction is rooted in evolutionary biology, hormonal fluctuations, and the roles that women have played throughout history. To truly understand the science of fasting and fat loss, one must delve deep into the specific metabolic nuances of the female body.

Historically, women have been gatherers, caregivers, and nurturers. From an evolutionary standpoint, the female body has been designed to ensure the survival of the species. This involves storing fat more efficiently, maintaining fertility, and providing sustenance for offspring. These roles have shaped the female metabolism in specific ways that influence how women process food, store fat, and respond to fasting.

Hormonal Symphny

At the heart of the female metabolism lies a complex interplay of hormones. These hormones fluctuate throughout the menstrual cycle and play a vital role in regulating metabolism, mood, and reproductive health.

Estrogen: Often referred to as the "female hormone," estrogen plays a crucial role in regulating fat storage and distribution. It promotes fat storage in the hips and thighs, which is thought to provide cushioning for pregnancy. Additionally, estrogen can increase insulin sensitivity, making it easier for women to utilize glucose for energy.

Progesterone: This hormone rises in the second half of the menstrual cycle. It has a calming effect and can increase the body's temperature, leading to slightly higher calorie burning. Progesterone also counteracts the effects of estrogen, ensuring a balance in the body.

Leptin: This hormone signals satiety to the brain. Interestingly, women generally have higher leptin levels than men, but they are also more resistant to its effects. This can lead to increased hunger and a greater propensity to store fat.

Ghrelin: Known as the "hunger hormone," ghrelin levels fluctuate in women based on their menstrual cycle. This can lead to varying levels of hunger throughout the month.

Understanding these hormonal fluctuations is essential when considering fasting and dietary strategies for women. For instance, during certain times of the menstrual cycle, women may benefit from higher carbohydrate intake, while at other times, they might respond better to a lower carbohydrate approach.

The Role of Body Fat

Women naturally have a higher percentage of body fat than men. This isn't just a matter of aesthetics; it's a biological necessity. Essential fat, which is the fat necessary to maintain life and reproductive functions, is higher in women. This fat plays a role in hormone production, especially hormones vital for reproduction.

Furthermore, the distribution of fat in women, primarily around the hips and thighs, serves evolutionary purposes. This pattern of fat storage provides protection and cushioning for the fetus during pregnancy. It also serves as an energy reserve for breastfeeding.

When considering fat loss strategies, it's important to understand that the female body is naturally inclined to hold onto fat reserves. This isn't a sign of metabolic dysfunction but rather a protective mechanism. However, with the right approach, women can optimize their metabolism for fat loss while respecting their body's natural inclinations.

Fasting and the Female Metabolism

While fasting offers a plethora of health benefits, its effects can vary based on gender. For women, the hormonal symphony that governs metabolism means that the response to fasting can be different.

For some women, intermittent fasting can lead to improved insulin sensitivity, enhanced fat burning, and even better hormonal balance. However, for others, especially when fasting is prolonged or too frequent, it can lead to hormonal imbalances, disrupted menstrual cycles, and fertility issues.

This doesn't mean that women should avoid fasting. Instead, it emphasizes the importance of a tailored approach. Women might benefit from shorter fasting windows or periodic fasting rather than daily restrictions. It's also crucial to pay attention to the body's signals. If fasting leads to mood disturbances, sleep issues, or menstrual irregularities, it might be time to reassess and modify the approach.

The Importance of Nutrition

For the female metabolism, what's consumed during eating windows is just as important as the fasting period. Nutrient-dense foods that provide essential vitamins and minerals can support hormonal health, boost metabolism, and ensure overall well-being.

Given the unique metabolic needs of women, especially concerning iron, calcium, and folate, a well-thought-out nutritional strategy is paramount. Emphasizing whole foods, healthy fats, lean proteins, and a colorful array of fruits and vegetables can support the metabolic processes and make fasting more effective and sustainable.

In conclusion, the female metabolism is a beautifully complex system shaped by evolution, biology, and hormonal interplay. It's a system designed for survival, reproduction, and nurturing. While this can present challenges in the realm of weight loss and metabolic optimization, with understanding and respect for this intricacy, women can harness their metabolic power. Through tailored fasting strategies, mindful nutrition, and an appreciation for the body's signals, women can achieve their health and weight loss goals while honoring their unique metabolic blueprint.

The Relationship Between Fasting, Fat Burning, and Female Hormones

The dance of hormones in the female body is intricate and delicate. Hormones dictate everything from mood to fertility, and understanding their role is crucial in the realm of health, fat burning, and fasting. As women embark on fasting regimens for health or weight loss, it's vital to appreciate how fasting impacts female hormones and, in turn, how these hormones influence the body's response to fasting.

Fasting: A Brief Overview

Fasting, at its core, is a period of abstaining from food. The duration can range from short intermittent fasting windows, such as 16 hours, to extended multi-day fasts. When a person fasts, the body undergoes a series of physiological changes. One of the primary shifts is the body's source of energy. In the absence of incoming glucose from food, the body taps into stored glycogen. When these reserves deplete, fat stores become the primary energy source, leading to fat burning and the production of ketones.

The Dance of Hormones During Fasting

As the body transitions from glucose burning to fat burning during a fast, a cascade of hormonal changes ensues:

Insulin: Fasting leads to lowered insulin levels. Insulin, the hormone responsible for shuttling glucose into cells, decreases when there's no incoming food. Lower insulin levels facilitate the breakdown of stored fat for energy.

Cortisol: Often referred to as the stress hormone, cortisol levels can increase during fasting. While this rise can enhance alertness and energy, prolonged elevated cortisol can have implications for female reproductive hormones.

Growth Hormone: Fasting stimulates the secretion of growth hormone, which aids in fat metabolism and muscle preservation. This hormone also has beneficial effects on collagen production, skin health, and overall longevity.

Norepinephrine: This neurotransmitter and hormone increases during fasting, boosting metabolism and facilitating fat burning.

Female Hormones and Their Dance with Fasting

While the hormones listed above play significant roles during fasting, it's the unique female hormones, primarily estrogen and progesterone, that require special attention in the context of fasting:

Estrogen: Fasting can influence estrogen levels in various ways. In the short term, fasting may lead to a slight increase in estrogen. However, prolonged fasting or frequent intermittent fasting can potentially decrease estrogen levels. This fluctuation can impact fat storage, mood, and even menstrual cycle regularity.

Progesterone: Progesterone levels can decrease with prolonged fasting. Since progesterone is essential for fertility and counteracts the effects of estrogen, this can lead to hormonal imbalances, mood disturbances, and irregular menstrual cycles.

Leptin and Ghrelin: These hunger hormones also interact uniquely with fasting in women. As mentioned previously, women have higher leptin levels, signaling satiety, but are more resistant to its effects. Fasting can further reduce leptin levels in women, potentially increasing hunger. Ghrelin, the hunger hormone, might spike more significantly in women during fasting, leading to increased appetite.

The Implications of Hormonal Changes

The interplay between fasting and female hormones is multifaceted. On the one hand, fasting can offer benefits like improved insulin sensitivity, enhanced fat burning, and cellular repair through processes like autophagy. On the other, if not done mindfully, fasting can disrupt the delicate hormonal balance in women.

Menstrual Cycle Irregularities: Prolonged or aggressive fasting can lead to missed periods or changes in menstrual cycle regularity. This is often due to the body perceiving fasting as a form of stress, potentially impacting reproductive capability.

Fertility: Reduced progesterone levels due to aggressive fasting can impact fertility. Since progesterone prepares the uterine lining for a fertilized egg, lower levels can make it harder to conceive.

Mood and Sleep: Hormonal fluctuations due to fasting can influence mood, leading to symptoms like irritability or depression. Sleep can also be impacted, with some women experiencing insomnia or disrupted sleep patterns.

Striking a Balance: Tailored Fasting for Women

Given the unique hormonal landscape of women, a one-size-fits-all approach to fasting may not be ideal. Instead, women can consider the following strategies:

Gentler Intermittent Fasting: Instead of aggressive fasting windows, women might benefit from shorter fasting periods, such as 12-14 hours. This provides a balance between the benefits of fasting without extreme hormonal shifts.

Cyclical Fasting: Aligning fasting with the menstrual cycle can be beneficial. For instance, during the follicular phase (the first half of the menstrual cycle), women might tolerate fasting better. In contrast, during the luteal phase (the second half), when energy needs are higher, shorter fasts or no fasting might be more appropriate.

Nutrient Timing: Paying attention to nutrient intake during eating windows is crucial. Emphasizing iron-rich foods, healthy fats, and adequate protein can support hormonal health and overall well-being.

Listening to the Body: Every woman is unique. Some might thrive on regular intermittent fasting, while others might feel better with periodic fasting. Paying attention to signals like energy levels, mood, sleep, and menstrual regularity can guide adjustments to fasting routines.

While fasting presents a powerful tool for health optimization and fat loss, its interplay with female hormones requires careful consideration. By understanding this relationship, women can harness the benefits of fasting while respecting and nurturing their unique hormonal landscape.

Common Misconceptions About Fasting and Female Health

In the realm of health and wellness, fasting has been both revered and misunderstood. As its popularity grows, so does the pool of information, often leading to misconceptions, especially concerning female health. Unraveling these misconceptions is crucial for women to make informed decisions about incorporating fasting into their lives.

Misconception 1: Fasting Always Leads to Starvation Mode

One of the most prevalent myths is that fasting sends the body into "starvation mode," slowing metabolism and causing the body to cling to its fat stores. While it's true that severe calorie restriction over extended periods can decrease metabolic rate, intermittent fasting does not produce the same effect. In fact, short-term fasting can boost metabolism by increasing norepinephrine levels. For women, the key is to ensure that when they do eat, they're consuming nutrient-dense foods that support overall health.

Misconception 2: Fasting Causes Muscle Loss in Women

The fear of muscle loss is another concern often voiced. The body is adaptive; during fasting, growth hormone levels rise, which protects muscle tissue. While prolonged fasting without adequate protein intake can lead to muscle loss, intermittent fasting, especially when combined with resistance training and proper nutrition, can preserve and even enhance muscle mass in women.

Misconception 3: All Women Will Experience Hormonal Imbalance from Fasting

While it's true that some women may experience hormonal shifts with aggressive or prolonged fasting, it's not a universal outcome. Many women practice intermittent fasting without any adverse effects on their menstrual cycle or hormonal health. Listening to one's body and making adjustments based on individual responses is essential.

Misconception 4: Fasting is Detrimental to Female Fertility

Concerns about fertility often arise when discussing fasting and women. While extreme weight loss or chronic caloric restriction can impact fertility, periodic intermittent fasting does not necessarily have this effect. In some cases, improving insulin sensitivity and reducing inflammation through fasting can actually enhance fertility. However, women trying to conceive should consult with a healthcare professional to determine the best approach for their individual needs.

Misconception 5: Fasting Will Make Women Fatigued and Unable to Function

Another common myth is that women will feel constantly tired and unable to carry out daily activities when fasting. In reality, many women report increased energy and mental clarity during fasting periods. This is due to the body switching from glucose to ketones as a primary energy source, which can provide a steady and sustained form of energy.

Misconception 6: Fasting Triggers Eating Disorders in Women

Concerns about fasting leading to eating disorders, especially in women, are valid. However, it's crucial to differentiate between mindful, intentional fasting and chronic caloric restriction or binge-purge behaviors. While fasting can be a therapeutic tool for health optimization, anyone with a history of eating disorders should approach it with caution and under professional guidance.

Misconception 7: Women Should Always Eat Small, Frequent Meals for Metabolism

The idea that women should graze throughout the day to "keep the metabolism active" is widespread. While there's nothing inherently wrong with eating small, frequent meals, it's not the only way to maintain or boost metabolism. Fasting, combined with periods of nutrient-dense eating, can be just as effective, if not more so, for metabolic health.

Misconception 8: Fasting Causes Hair Loss in Women

Hair loss can be alarming, and some women have reported hair thinning or loss after starting a fasting regimen. It's essential to understand that significant dietary changes can cause temporary hair shedding, known as telogen effluvium. This is not exclusive to fasting and can occur with any major dietary shift. Ensuring adequate protein and micronutrient intake during eating windows can support hair health.

Misconception 9: Fasting is the Same for Women of All Ages

A woman's metabolic and hormonal needs shift throughout her life. What works for a woman in her 20s might not be suitable for a woman in her 50s. Factors like menstrual cycle, perimenopause, and post-menopause status can influence how a woman responds to fasting. Tailoring fasting regimens to life stages is crucial.

Misconception 10: Fasting Means Completely Avoiding Food

The term "fasting" often conjures images of abstaining from all food for extended periods. In reality, there are many fasting protocols, from time-restricted eating to alternate-day fasting, to modified fasts that include small amounts of food. Women can choose a method that aligns with their health goals and lifestyle.

As fasting continues to gain traction in the health community, it's essential for women to separate fact from fiction. The key lies in understanding the science, listening to one's body, and being willing to adapt and adjust based on individual experiences and needs.

As the journey through the science of fasting and fat loss continues, the subsequent sections will provide a deeper dive into practical strategies, insights, and empowering information to help each woman navigate her unique path to health and freedom.

Setting the Stage: What to Expect in Your Feminine Fasting Journey

Embarking on a fasting journey is akin to setting forth on a voyage of self-discovery. Each woman's experience is unique, shaped by her biology, lifestyle, and personal goals. While fasting has universal principles, the nuances of the feminine body add layers of complexity and wonder. Knowing what to expect can provide clarity, set the stage for success, and foster a deeper connection with one's body.

1. Initial Reactions and Adaptations

The first foray into fasting often comes with a set of physical and emotional reactions. As the body shifts from a glucose-fueled system to one that burns fat, some common experiences include:

Hunger Pangs: These are natural, especially during the initial days. Over time, as the body becomes accustomed to fasting, these sensations often diminish.

Energy Fluctuations: Some women report feeling a surge of energy, while others might feel temporarily fatigued as their metabolism adjusts.

Mental Clarity: The brain thrives on ketones, which are produced during fasting. This can lead to enhanced focus and clarity.

Emotional Responses: Fasting is not just a physical journey. It can bring up emotions related to food, body image, and self-worth. Being prepared for this emotional landscape is crucial.

2. Hormonal Shifts and Their Implications

As discussed in previous sections, fasting can influence female hormones. While many women sail through fasting without any issues, others might notice:

Menstrual Cycle Changes: Some women report changes in cycle length, flow, or even missed periods. Monitoring these changes and adjusting fasting routines can help.

Mood Variations: Hormonal fluctuations can influence mood. Being aware of this can aid in navigating any emotional waves with grace.

Changes in Hunger and Satiety: Hormones like ghrelin and leptin, which regulate hunger and fullness, can be influenced by fasting. Over time, many women find that their hunger cues become more regulated.

3. Physical Transformations

Beyond the internal changes, fasting can lead to visible physical transformations:

Weight Loss: Many women turn to fasting for its weight loss benefits. While weight loss can be a natural outcome, it's essential to approach it with a holistic mindset, focusing on overall health.

Improved Skin Health: Autophagy, a cellular cleanup process activated during fasting, can lead to clearer and more radiant skin.

Enhanced Digestion: Giving the digestive system a break can improve gut health, reduce bloating, and alleviate some digestive disorders.

4. The Evolution of Tastes and Preferences

An unexpected yet delightful aspect of fasting is the evolution of one's palate:

Reduced Cravings: Over time, many women notice a reduction in cravings, especially for sugary or highly processed foods.

Savoring Simplicity: As the body becomes attuned to natural hunger and satiety cues, there's often a newfound appreciation for simple, nourishing foods.

Intuitive Eating: With regular fasting, many women find that they develop a more intuitive relationship with food, gravitating towards what their body truly needs.

5. The Power of Flexibility

One of the pillars of a successful feminine fasting journey is flexibility. Life events, menstrual cycles, and personal commitments can all influence one's fasting routine:

Adapting to Life's Rhythms: Whether it's adjusting fasting windows during specific phases of the menstrual cycle or accommodating social events, the ability to adapt is crucial.

Listening and Adjusting: The body's signals are paramount. If something feels off, or if there are signs of hormonal imbalance, it might be time to reassess and modify the fasting approach.

6. The Deepening Connection with Self

Perhaps one of the most profound aspects of the feminine fasting journey is the deepening connection with oneself:

Body Awareness: Fasting can heighten body awareness, tuning women into subtle signals and cues that might have been overlooked before.

Emotional Exploration: Without the constant cycle of eating and digestion, there's space for introspection. This can lead to profound emotional and spiritual growth.

Empowerment: Taking control of one's health, understanding the body's rhythms, and harnessing the power of fasting can be incredibly empowering for women.

As the chapters unfold in this guide, the exploration will dive deeper, providing tools, insights, and strategies to support each woman on her unique fasting voyage. The journey is one of empowerment, transformation, and a celebration of the feminine body in all its wonder.

3

Hormonal Harmony through Fasting

The Estrogen-Fasting Connection

Estrogen is often colloquially referred to as the "female hormone," though it plays significant roles in bodies of all genders. In females, its ebb and flow shape the menstrual cycle, influence mood, modulate metabolism, and even impact cognitive function. Given its pervasive influence, understanding how fasting interacts with estrogen is paramount for women considering this health practice.

Estrogen: A Brief Overview

To appreciate the estrogen-fasting connection, a foundational understanding of estrogen's role in the body is essential:

Reproductive Health: Estrogen prepares the uterus for a potential pregnancy after ovulation, thickening its lining to receive a fertilized egg.

Bone Health: This hormone aids in the absorption of calcium and the production of bone-building cells, ensuring skeletal strength.

Heart Health: Estrogen supports the health of blood vessels and helps regulate cholesterol levels.

Brain Function: Beyond its role in reproduction, estrogen influences mood, memory, and even pain perception.

Given its multifaceted roles, any intervention that impacts estrogen levels, such as fasting, must be approached with knowledge and care.

Fasting's Impact on Estrogen Levels

At first glance, fasting and estrogen might seem unrelated. However, the relationship between nutrition, metabolic health, and hormonal balance is intricate:

Liver Function and Estrogen Metabolism: The liver plays a pivotal role in metabolizing and excreting excess estrogen. Fasting enhances liver function, facilitating the efficient processing of hormones. This can help balance estrogen levels and reduce symptoms of estrogen dominance, a condition where there's a relative excess of estrogen compared to progesterone.

Body Fat and Estrogen Production: Adipose tissue, or body fat, is not just an inert storage depot. It's an active endocrine organ that produces estrogen. Fasting promotes fat burning, reducing the total amount of estrogen-producing tissue. This can be especially relevant for postmenopausal women, where adipose tissue becomes a primary estrogen source.

Insulin Sensitivity and Hormonal Balance: Insulin, the hormone responsible for managing blood sugar, has a complex relationship with other hormones, including estrogen. Improved insulin sensitivity, often achieved through fasting, can positively influence estrogen balance.

The Dual-Edged Sword: Potential Benefits and Considerations

While the estrogen-fasting connection offers potential benefits, it also presents considerations to ensure hormonal harmony:

Benefits:

Reduced Symptoms of Estrogen Dominance: Symptoms like bloating, mood swings, irregular periods, and breast tenderness can be mitigated with improved estrogen metabolism through fasting.

Improved Reproductive Health: For women with conditions like polycystic ovary syndrome (PCOS), characterized by hormonal imbalances, fasting can aid in restoring hormonal harmony.

Enhanced Cognitive Function: Given estrogen's role in brain health, optimizing its levels through fasting can lead to better mood, memory, and cognitive agility.

Considerations:

Excessive Estrogen Drop: While balancing elevated estrogen is beneficial, excessively lowering it can have repercussions. Estrogen plays protective roles in heart health, bone density, and more. Women need to strike a balance to ensure they're not depriving their bodies of this vital hormone.

Potential Menstrual Irregularities: Any intervention that significantly impacts hormones can influence menstrual cycle regularity. Some women might experience changes in cycle length, flow, or even skipped periods. Monitoring and adapting fasting practices can help navigate these changes.

Interactions with Hormonal Medications: Women on hormonal medications, including birth control or hormone replacement therapy, should be aware of potential interactions. Fasting can influence how the body processes these medications, impacting their efficacy.

Tailoring Fasting Practices for Optimal Estrogen Balance

The key to harnessing the benefits of fasting for estrogen balance lies in individualization:

Start Slowly: For those new to fasting, gradual introduction allows the body time to adjust, reducing potential disruptions to estrogen balance.

Monitor and Adjust: Keeping track of symptoms, menstrual cycle changes, and overall well-being can provide insights into how fasting impacts estrogen. Adjustments in fasting duration or frequency can be made based on these observations.

Supportive Nutrition: During eating windows, emphasizing foods that support liver health and hormonal balance can enhance fasting's benefits. Cruciferous vegetables, for instance, aid in estrogen metabolism.

The estrogen-fasting connection provides a window into the intricate dance of female physiology. By understanding and respecting this relationship, women can leverage fasting as a powerful tool for hormonal harmony, overall health, and well-being. As this chapter unfolds, the exploration will further delve into other hormonal interactions, offering insights and strategies to create a symphony of hormonal balance through fasting.

Insulin Sensitivity and Fasting

In the intricate world of hormones, insulin stands out as a pivotal player, especially in the context of metabolic health. Often associated with diabetes, insulin's role extends far beyond blood sugar regulation. It influences fat storage, interacts with other hormones, and plays a role in overall energy balance. Within this spectrum, fasting emerges as a potent tool to modulate insulin sensitivity, offering profound implications for health and well-being.

Understanding Insulin: More Than Just Blood Sugar

Insulin is a hormone produced by the pancreas in response to elevated blood sugar, primarily after meals:

Glucose Management: Insulin's primary role is to facilitate the uptake of glucose into cells, ensuring that tissues receive the energy they need while maintaining blood sugar stability.

Fat Storage: Insulin also promotes the storage of excess energy as fat, ensuring reserves for future use.

Protein Synthesis: Beyond glucose and fat, insulin plays a role in muscle growth, promoting protein synthesis and inhibiting its breakdown.

Given these multifaceted roles, it's evident that optimal insulin function is crucial for metabolic health.

The Spectrum of Insulin Sensitivity

Insulin sensitivity refers to how responsive cells are to insulin's signals:

High Insulin Sensitivity: Cells respond well to insulin, efficiently taking up glucose from the bloodstream. This is the desired state, as it ensures efficient energy use and stable blood sugar levels.

Insulin Resistance: Over time, due to factors like chronic overeating, sedentary lifestyle, or genetic predisposition, cells can become less responsive to insulin. The pancreas compensates by producing more insulin, leading to elevated insulin levels. This state is associated with a host of health issues,

including type 2 diabetes, cardiovascular disease, and even some cancers.
Fasting's Role in Modulating Insulin Sensitivity

Given the challenges associated with insulin resistance, strategies to enhance insulin sensitivity are of paramount importance. Here's where fasting enters the scene:

Reduced Blood Sugar and Insulin Levels: Naturally, in the absence of food, blood sugar levels stabilize, and there's reduced need for insulin. Over time, this reduces the pancreas's workload and allows insulin levels to normalize.

Cellular Repair and Autophagy: Fasting triggers autophagy, a cellular "clean-up" process. This process can rejuvenate insulin receptors on cell surfaces, enhancing their responsiveness to insulin.

Fat Loss: Excess visceral fat, the kind stored around organs, is linked to insulin resistance. Fasting promotes fat burning, reducing visceral fat and thereby improving insulin sensitivity.

Implications for Female Health

The insulin-fasting connection holds specific implications for female health:

Polycystic Ovary Syndrome (PCOS): One of the hallmarks of PCOS is insulin resistance. Fasting, by improving insulin sensitivity, offers potential benefits for women with this condition, including improved menstrual regularity and fertility.

Pregnancy and Gestational Diabetes: Insulin resistance increases during pregnancy, making gestational diabetes a risk for many women. While fasting is not typically recommended during pregnancy, understanding and managing insulin sensitivity before conception can reduce risks.

Menopause: The transition to menopause can bring about changes in insulin sensitivity. Fasting offers a tool to manage these shifts, supporting metabolic health during this life phase.

Strategies and Considerations

Harnessing fasting for insulin sensitivity requires a nuanced approach:

Gradual Introduction: For those new to fasting, a slow introduction, such as 12-hour overnight fasts, can provide the body time to adjust.

Hydration: Drinking ample water supports the kidneys in flushing out excess glucose, enhancing fasting's benefits.

Balanced Break-Fast: When ending a fast, it's crucial to consume balanced meals. Combining protein, healthy fats, and fiber-rich carbohydrates can ensure sustained energy and avoid rapid blood sugar spikes.

Monitor Blood Sugar: Those with diabetes or on medications that influence blood sugar should monitor levels closely and consult with healthcare providers before embarking on fasting regimens.

The interplay between insulin sensitivity and fasting offers a window into the body's remarkable adaptability. By harnessing the benefits of fasting, women can optimize insulin function, promoting metabolic health, vitality, and hormonal harmony. As this exploration continues, subsequent sections will delve deeper into other hormonal interactions with fasting, weaving together a tapestry of understanding and strategies for holistic well-being.

Impact of Fasting on Thyroid Hormones

The thyroid gland, a butterfly-shaped organ nestled in the neck, plays a pivotal role in regulating metabolism, energy production, and overall vitality. The hormones it secretes influence every cell, tissue, and organ in the body. Given this widespread impact, understanding how fasting influences thyroid hormones is crucial for those seeking to harness the benefits of fasting without compromising thyroid health.

Thyroid Hormones: A Primer

To comprehend the fasting-thyroid connection, a foundational understanding of thyroid hormones and their functions is essential:

Thyroxine (T4): This is the primary hormone produced by the thyroid gland. It's a prohormone, meaning it's inactive in this form and needs to be converted to its active counterpart.

Triiodothyronine (T3): Derived from T4, T3 is the active thyroid hormone that exerts metabolic effects throughout the body.

Thyroid Stimulating Hormone (TSH): Produced by the pituitary gland in the brain, TSH signals the thyroid gland to produce and release thyroid hormones.

Together, these hormones regulate metabolic rate, heart function, digestion, mood, and more.

Fasting's Interplay with Thyroid Hormones

Fasting introduces a state of reduced caloric intake, signaling the body to make various metabolic adaptations. Among these, alterations in thyroid hormone levels can occur:

1. **T3 Reduction:** During prolonged fasting, levels of the active thyroid hormone T3 may decrease. This is a natural adaptation, as the body aims to conserve energy during periods of reduced caloric intake.
2. **T4 Stability:** The levels of T4, the inactive thyroid hormone, generally remain stable during short-term fasting. However, prolonged fasting might influence T4 levels, though the effects can be variable.
3. **TSH Fluctuations:** The response of TSH to fasting is complex. In some individuals, TSH may increase, while in others, it remains unchanged or decreases.

Implications for Metabolic Health

The changes in thyroid hormones during fasting have specific implications:

Metabolic Slowdown: A reduction in T3 levels can lead to a temporary slowdown in metabolism. This is the body's way of conserving energy during periods of limited caloric intake.

Thermogenesis: Thyroid hormones play a role in body temperature regulation. Altered levels during fasting might influence the body's ability to generate heat.

Mood and Cognition: Given the role of thyroid hormones in brain function, changes in their levels during fasting can influence mood, alertness, and cognitive capabilities.

The Gender Lens: Fasting and Thyroid Health in Women

The interplay between fasting and thyroid hormones holds specific considerations for women:

Menstrual Cycle: Thyroid hormones interact with reproductive hormones. Changes in thyroid function can influence menstrual cycle regularity.

Fertility: Optimal thyroid function is crucial for fertility. Women considering pregnancy should be mindful of any fasting regimen's impact on thyroid health.

Bone Health: Thyroid hormones influence bone metabolism. Prolonged fasting and its effects on thyroid function could have implications for bone density, especially in postmenopausal women.

Navigating Fasting for Optimal Thyroid Health

Harnessing fasting's benefits while ensuring thyroid health requires a balanced approach:

1. **Short-Term Fasting:** For those concerned about thyroid health, sticking to shorter fasting windows, such as 12 to 16 hours, might be preferable.
2. **Nutrient Intake:** During eating windows, emphasizing foods rich in iodine, selenium, and zinc can support thyroid function. These include seafood, nuts, and seeds.
3. **Monitoring:** Regularly checking thyroid hormone levels, especially if one engages in prolonged or frequent fasting, can provide insights into how fasting impacts thyroid health.
4. **Holistic View:** Beyond just hormone levels, monitoring symptoms like energy, mood, skin health, and body temperature can offer a comprehensive view of thyroid function during fasting.

The relationship between fasting and thyroid hormones offers insights into the body's adaptability and resilience. By understanding this dynamic and navigating fasting practices with awareness and care, individuals can achieve metabolic health, hormonal harmony, and holistic well-being. As this exploration continues, subsequent sections will delve into the nuances of other hormonal pathways, weaving a rich tapestry of understanding and guidance for those seeking harmony through fasting.

Progesterone and Fasting: A Delicate Balance

While estrogen often steals the limelight in discussions about female hormones, progesterone is its lesser-known but equally vital counterpart. Integral to menstrual cycle regulation, mood balance, and pregnancy, progesterone plays crucial roles in female physiology. As fasting emerges as a tool for hormonal optimization, understanding its interplay with progesterone becomes essential for women seeking to achieve hormonal harmony.

The Role of Progesterone

To comprehend the nuances of the progesterone-fasting relationship, one must first grasp progesterone's functions:

Menstrual Cycle Regulation: After ovulation, the ruptured follicle transforms into the corpus luteum, which produces progesterone. This hormone prepares the uterine lining for a potential embryo implantation.

Pregnancy Support: If an embryo implants, progesterone helps maintain the uterine lining for a fertilized egg to grow.

Mood Modulation: Progesterone has a calming effect on the brain and can influence mood and anxiety levels.

Bone Health: This hormone aids in the bone-building process, supporting skeletal health.

Fasting's Influence on Progesterone Levels

Diving into the realm of fasting and its effects on progesterone reveals a multifaceted dynamic:

Short-Term Fasting: Brief fasting periods, such as intermittent fasting, generally have minimal impact on progesterone levels for most women. However, individual responses can vary, and some might experience changes in menstrual cycle length or intensity.

Prolonged Fasting: Extended fasting durations can lead to significant caloric and nutrient deficits, potentially impacting ovulation. Without ovulation, the corpus luteum doesn't form, leading to reduced progesterone production.

Stress and Progesterone: Fasting is a form of physiological stress. The body's response to stress includes the release of cortisol, a hormone produced in the adrenal glands. Chronic elevation of cortisol can divert precursors away from progesterone production, leading to lower progesterone levels.

Implications for Female Health

Understanding how fasting impacts progesterone is pivotal given its broad influence on female health:

Menstrual Irregularities: As noted, changes in progesterone levels can affect the menstrual cycle. Some women might experience shorter cycles, lighter periods, or even missed cycles, depending on the fasting regimen and individual physiology.

Mood and Well-being: Given progesterone's role in mood modulation, changes in its levels can influence emotional well-being. Some women might feel more relaxed, while others could experience mood swings or heightened anxiety.

Fertility Considerations: Progesterone is crucial for preparing the uterus for pregnancy and supporting it in the early stages. Women looking to conceive should approach fasting with caution and be attentive to its potential impact on progesterone and overall fertility.

Strategies for Maintaining Progesterone Balance

For those keen on integrating fasting into their lifestyle while ensuring optimal progesterone levels, several strategies can be employed:

Gradual Introduction: As with any significant lifestyle change, easing into fasting can allow the body to adjust gradually, potentially mitigating abrupt hormonal shifts.

Nutrient-Rich Eating Windows: Emphasizing foods rich in nutrients that support progesterone production, such as vitamin B6, zinc, and magnesium, can be beneficial. These include poultry, seafood, nuts, and leafy greens.

Manage Stress: Incorporating relaxation techniques, such as meditation, deep breathing exercises, or gentle yoga, can help manage cortisol levels and support hormonal balance.

Regular Monitoring: Keeping track of menstrual cycles, mood, and overall well-being can offer insights into how fasting impacts progesterone levels. Adjusting fasting practices based on these observations can help achieve hormonal harmony.

The delicate dance between progesterone and fasting underscores the body's intricate hormonal symphony. Recognizing the nuances of this relationship and navigating fasting with knowledge and intention can empower women to harness its benefits while maintaining hormonal equilibrium. As the exploration of hormonal harmony through fasting continues, subsequent sections will delve deeper into other facets of this fascinating journey, offering insights and guidance for those seeking balance, well-being, and holistic health.

Hormonal Fluctuations Throughout the Menstrual Cycle and Fasting Strategies

The menstrual cycle, a symphony of hormonal fluctuations, is a profound reflection of a woman's reproductive health. As estrogen and progesterone ebb and flow, they influence mood, energy, metabolism, and more. Introducing fasting into this dynamic landscape requires understanding and respect for these hormonal rhythms. Crafting fasting strategies tailored to different phases of the menstrual cycle can optimize benefits while honoring the body's innate wisdom.

The Four Phases of the Menstrual Cycle

To navigate fasting throughout the menstrual cycle, one must first understand its four distinct phases:

Menstrual Phase (Days 1-5): This is the bleeding phase, marking the beginning of a new cycle. Estrogen and progesterone levels are at their lowest, leading to the shedding of the uterine lining.

Follicular Phase (Days 1-13): Overlapping with the menstrual phase, this phase is characterized by rising estrogen levels as follicles in the ovaries mature, preparing for ovulation.

Ovulatory Phase (Days 14-16): Estrogen peaks, leading to the release of a mature egg from the ovary, signaling the body's readiness for fertilization.

Luteal Phase (Days 15-28): After ovulation, the ruptured follicle becomes the corpus luteum, producing progesterone. This phase prepares the uterus for potential pregnancy.

Fasting Strategies Tailored to the Menstrual Cycle

With an understanding of the hormonal landscape throughout the menstrual cycle, fasting can be tailored to support and harmonize with these rhythms:

Menstrual Phase:

Energy might be lower during this phase, making it a less ideal time for extended fasts.

Gentle, shorter fasts, if desired, can be integrated, ensuring adequate iron intake during eating windows to compensate for menstrual blood loss.

Hydration is crucial to support the body in flushing out waste and preventing bloating.

Follicular Phase:

As estrogen rises, energy levels and mood often improve, making this an optimal phase for longer fasts.

The body is more insulin-sensitive, enhancing the benefits of fasting for metabolic health.

Engaging in more vigorous physical activity during fasting windows can be supported by the surge in energy.

Ovulatory Phase:

With peak estrogen levels, energy is typically at its highest, supporting more extended or frequent fasts.

However, it's essential to ensure adequate caloric and nutrient intake, as the body prepares for potential pregnancy.

Luteal Phase:

As progesterone dominates, body temperature rises, and energy needs might increase.

Cravings can be more pronounced, making strict fasting more challenging. Opting for a more relaxed fasting window or incorporating nutrient-dense snacks can be beneficial.

Prioritizing foods rich in magnesium and B vitamins can support mood and energy.

Individual Variations and Listening to the Body

While the above strategies offer a general roadmap, it's paramount to recognize individual variations:

Cycle Length: Not all women have a textbook 28-day cycle. Adjusting fasting strategies to one's unique cycle length is crucial.

Symptom Management: For women with menstrual symptoms like PMS or cramps, fasting might either alleviate or exacerbate symptoms. Monitoring and adjusting based on personal experience is essential.

Body Signals: Above all, tuning into the body's signals is the most potent guide. Feelings of extreme fatigue, persistent hunger, or mood disturbances might indicate the need for adjustments in fasting practices.

The intricate dance of hormones throughout the menstrual cycle offers a window into the body's profound rhythms. By tailoring fasting strategies to these rhythms, women can harness the benefits of fasting while respecting and supporting their reproductive health. As the exploration of hormonal harmony through fasting concludes, it's evident that the journey is one of deep respect, understanding, and alignment with the body's wisdom.

This alignment paves the way for holistic health, vitality, and a deepened connection with one's body and being.

33

4

Tailoring Fasts for Phases of the Menstrual Cycle

Menstrual phase: Gentle fasting

The menstrual cycle is a natural process that each woman undergoes monthly. During this period, a woman's body undergoes various hormonal shifts which can influence energy levels, mood, metabolism, and more. Recognizing and understanding these shifts can aid in optimizing one's fasting strategy to align with the body's unique needs during each phase. The menstrual phase, which is the beginning of the cycle, is when bleeding occurs. This is a time when the body is releasing the uterine lining. Given the delicate nature of this period, it's crucial to approach fasting with sensitivity and gentleness.

The Science Behind Menstrual Phase

In the menstrual phase, there are significant drops in the levels of both estrogen and progesterone, the primary female hormones. The decline in these hormones is what causes the uterine lining to shed, leading to menstruation. This period can last from 3 to 7 days for most women.

The drop in hormones, particularly estrogen, can lead to reduced energy levels, mood swings, and a heightened sensitivity to pain. Metabolically, there is a decrease in basal metabolic rate (BMR) which means the body is burning fewer calories at rest than in other phases of the cycle. Digestion can slow, leading to bloating, and there's an increased demand for iron due to blood loss.

Why Gentle Fasting?

Given the physical and emotional vulnerabilities associated with this phase, it's wise to avoid extreme or prolonged fasting. Instead, a gentle approach to fasting can be beneficial. Gentle fasting can mean shorter fast durations, ensuring adequate hydration, and consuming specific nutrients that support the body during this time.

Gentle fasting during the menstrual phase is not about pushing the body to its limits but about honoring its processes and supporting its needs. Fasting should not feel punitive but rather like a practice of self-care.

Benefits of Gentle Fasting During Menstrual Phase

Detoxification: The menstrual phase is a natural detox period for women. Gentle fasting can aid the body's detoxification process without overburdening it. It's a period of renewal and shedding, and a mild fast can enhance this.

Energy Conservation: As the body's energy levels might be lower during this phase, gentle fasting can aid in conserving energy. By giving the digestive system a rest, even if it's just for a shorter period, it allows the body to allocate energy to other vital processes.

Hormonal Balance: Even though estrogen and progesterone levels drop during this phase, gentle fasting can help balance other hormones like insulin, which can have positive effects on mood and energy.

Digestive Relief: With digestion being slower during the menstrual phase, gentle fasting can provide the digestive system with a much-needed break, potentially reducing bloating and discomfort.

How to Practice Gentle Fasting During the Menstrual Phase

Duration: Consider shorter fasts, like the 12:12 method where you eat within a 12-hour window and fast for the next 12. This ensures you're still giving your body a break but not pushing it too hard.

Hydration: Drink plenty of water. Considering the blood loss, it's vital to stay hydrated. You can also incorporate herbal teas that are known to support menstrual health like raspberry leaf or chamomile.

Nutrient Intake: Prioritize iron-rich foods during your eating windows to compensate for the loss during menstruation. Foods like leafy greens, lentils, and certain meats can be beneficial. Also, consider foods rich in magnesium to help with cramps and Vitamin B6 for mood regulation.

Listen to Your Body: The most important thing during this phase (and indeed, all phases) is to tune into your body's signals. If you feel faint, overly fatigued, or just "off" in any way, it might be best to break your fast and consume some nourishing food.

Potential Challenges and How to Address Them

1. **Cravings:** Due to the hormonal shifts, you might experience increased cravings, especially for carbs and sweets. Instead of succumbing to unhealthy choices, try consuming complex carbohydrates like whole grains or sweet vegetables like sweet potatoes. These can satisfy cravings while still being nutritious.
2. **Fatigue:** This is common due to the drop in estrogen. If you feel overly tired, consider shortening your fasting window even further or taking a break from fasting altogether for a day or two.
3. **Emotional Sensitivity:** With the hormonal shifts can come mood swings. During your fasting, make time for self-care. This could be in the form of meditation, journaling, or even just ensuring you get enough sleep.

The menstrual phase is a time of renewal and letting go. It's a period where the body is undergoing significant internal processes, and it's essential to support these processes in the best way possible. Gentle fasting, when done with awareness and care, can be a powerful tool during this time, not just for detoxification and rest but as a practice of self-compassion and attunement to one's body.

While the menstrual phase has its unique considerations, so too do the other phases of the menstrual cycle. As we delve further into these phases, it becomes clear that each phase offers its opportunities and challenges in the realm of fasting. The key lies in understanding these nuances and tailoring one's fasting regimen accordingly.

Follicular phase: Fueling fertility

Following the menstrual phase, the follicular phase marks the beginning of the ovulation cycle, setting the stage for potential fertility. The body undergoes a series of transformations with the primary goal of preparing an egg for fertilization. The follicular phase is characterized by an increase in both energy levels and mood, courtesy of the rising estrogen levels. This presents a unique window of opportunity for a different approach to fasting, one that focuses on fueling fertility.

Understanding the Follicular Phase

The follicular phase commences on the first day of the menstrual cycle and lasts until ovulation begins, typically around day 14. This phase sees a surge in the follicle-stimulating hormone (FSH), which stimulates the growth of 5-20 small sacs in the ovaries, each containing an immature egg. As the phase progresses, only one egg dominates and matures, ready for ovulation.

Simultaneously, the endometrium or the lining of the uterus begins to thicken, preparing itself for a potential implantation of a fertilized egg. This phase is marked by an increase in estrogen, which boosts energy, elevates mood, and may enhance cognitive abilities.

Redefining Fasting in the Follicular Phase

The follicular phase, with its heightened energy and mood, offers a prime opportunity to capitalize on these advantages. As such, the focus shifts from gentle fasting to a method that fuels fertility and harnesses the natural energy surge.

Advantages of Fasting During the Follicular Phase

Enhanced Metabolic Flexibility: As the body experiences higher energy levels, fasting can promote metabolic flexibility, allowing the body to efficiently switch between using carbohydrates and fats as energy sources.

Boosted Cognitive Abilities: With increased estrogen levels, cognitive function, and memory may see improvement. Fasting, known for its neuroprotective benefits, can potentially amplify these effects.

Optimized Nutrient Absorption: Fasting can improve gut health, leading to better absorption of nutrients, vital for the fertility process.

Reinforced Detoxification: The body's natural detoxification processes get a boost, ensuring a conducive environment for fertility.

Strategies for Fasting During the Follicular Phase

Duration: Given the elevated energy levels, one might consider slightly longer fasts, such as the 16:8 method, where an 8-hour eating window is followed by a 16-hour fast. This approach can capitalize on the body's natural rhythm during this phase.

Hydration: As always, hydration remains crucial. Green teas can be beneficial, given their antioxidant properties, potentially supporting egg quality.

Nutrient Intake: Emphasize protein-rich foods to support the growing follicles. Foods like lean meats, legumes, and eggs can be beneficial. Zinc and Vitamin D also play crucial roles in fertility; consider foods like pumpkin seeds, mushrooms, and fortified dairy.

Incorporate Movement: With the increased energy, combine fasting with light exercises like walking or yoga. This promotes better blood circulation, potentially aiding the fertility process.

Challenges and Solutions in the Follicular Phase

1. **Overexertion:** While the increased energy is a boon, it's easy to overextend oneself. It's vital to listen to the body and not push too hard, even if energy levels suggest otherwise.
2. **Possible Dehydration:** Longer fasts might lead to dehydration. Ensure regular water intake and include electrolyte-rich drinks if needed.

3. Managing Hunger Pangs: With an active metabolism, hunger might strike more frequently. Opt for nutrient-dense snacks during eating windows, focusing on proteins and healthy fats for satiety.

The follicular phase, in all its dynamism, represents a period of preparation and potential. Recognizing and tapping into its unique attributes can shape a fasting protocol that not only complements the body's processes but also maximizes the inherent benefits of the phase.

Following the follicular phase, the body transitions into the ovulation phase, characterized by its distinct set of hormonal changes and physiological responses. Just as the follicular phase demanded a unique approach to fasting, so too does the ovulation phase, underscoring the need for adaptability and keen awareness of one's body throughout the menstrual cycle.

Ovulation phase: Balancing act

The ovulation phase is a pinnacle moment in the menstrual cycle. It's a short, yet significant window where the mature egg is released from the ovary, traveling down the fallopian tube, available for fertilization. Estrogen peaks, leading to a surge in the luteinizing hormone (LH) that triggers ovulation. It's a period of heightened fertility and embodies a complex interplay of hormones. Fasting during this phase demands a keen understanding and a balanced approach, hence aptly termed the "balancing act."

Deciphering the Ovulation Phase

Spanning just about 3-4 days, the ovulation phase typically occurs around the middle of the menstrual cycle, between days 14 and 17 for many women. It's a period when the body is most fertile. The estrogen peak during this phase boosts energy, mood, and libido. The cervical mucus becomes clearer and stretchy, signaling the body's readiness for potential conception.

However, the spike in estrogen also means increased insulin sensitivity. This is a crucial aspect to note when considering fasting during ovulation, as it affects how the body processes glucose.

The Fasting Paradigm in the Ovulation Phase

Given the complex hormonal landscape during ovulation, fasting requires a balanced, measured approach. It's neither about aggressive fasting nor complete abstinence but striking the right equilibrium.

Perks of Fasting During Ovulation

Optimized Energy Utilization: With heightened insulin sensitivity, the body becomes more efficient in using glucose, providing stable energy levels. Fasting can further fine-tune this energy utilization.

Mood Elevation: Fasting is known to boost certain neurotransmitters like serotonin, which when combined with the natural mood enhancement from estrogen, can lead to an overall positive disposition.

Support for Reproductive Health: Fasting can aid in cellular repair processes, potentially benefiting the reproductive organs.

Enhanced Cognitive Clarity: The combined effects of estrogen and the brain benefits from fasting can lead to sharper cognition and improved focus.

Approach to Fasting During the Ovulation Phase

Duration: Given the increased insulin sensitivity, it's advisable to opt for moderate fasts. The 14:10 method, a 14-hour fast followed by a 10-hour eating window, can be effective.

Hydration: Stay well-hydrated to support the cervical mucus production, vital during this phase. Infusions with cucumber or mint can be refreshing and supportive.

Nutrient Intake: Prioritize foods that stabilize blood sugar levels, given the insulin sensitivity. Incorporate whole grains, lean proteins, and healthy fats. Omega-3 rich foods like flaxseeds, chia seeds, and fish can support hormonal balance.

Gentle Exercise: Engage in moderate activities like brisk walking or cycling. It not only aids blood circulation but can also keep mood swings at bay.

Navigating Challenges in the Ovulation Phase

1. **Elevated Hunger:** The body might signal increased hunger during ovulation. Address this by consuming fiber-rich foods that promote satiety, like legumes and vegetables.
2. **Mood Fluctuations:** Even though mood is generally elevated, some women might experience mood dips. Ensure a nourishing diet and consider practices like meditation or deep breathing exercises for emotional balance.
3. **Over Sensitivity to Caffeine:** The body might react more strongly to stimulants like caffeine. It's prudent to reduce caffeine intake or opt for alternatives like herbal teas.

The ovulation phase, with its intricate hormonal dance, underscores the need for a delicate balance in fasting practices. It's about harnessing the natural vitality of this phase, amplifying its advantages, and ensuring that the body's fertility potential is not compromised.

With ovulation culminating, the menstrual cycle advances to the luteal phase, a period of preparation and potential anticipation. Just like its predecessors, the luteal phase presents its unique set of attributes and challenges, emphasizing the ever-evolving nature of the female body and the necessity for adaptive fasting strategies.

Luteal phase: Prepping for the fast

The luteal phase is a period of anticipation. Following ovulation, the body prepares itself for a potential pregnancy. If fertilization does not occur, it prepares for menstruation. The phase is characterized by the dominance of progesterone, a hormone that signals the uterus to thicken its lining in anticipation of a fertilized egg. This shift from the estrogen-dominant ovulation phase means a change in energy, mood, and appetite. Therefore, the approach to fasting during this time requires a focus on prepping the body for the menstrual phase, making it aptly titled "prepping for the fast."

The Luteal Phase Unveiled
The luteal phase typically lasts for about 14 days, starting after ovulation and ending just before menstruation. As the corpus luteum releases progesterone, body temperature rises slightly. If fertilization does not occur, the corpus luteum degenerates, leading to a drop in progesterone and eventually menstruation.

Many women notice changes in their mood, energy, and appetite during this phase. Some experience symptoms of premenstrual syndrome (PMS), which includes bloating, mood swings, irritability, and cravings.

Fasting Dynamics in the Luteal Phase
Given the body's preparation either for pregnancy or menstruation, the luteal phase requires a supportive and nourishing approach to fasting.

Benefits of Fasting in the Luteal Phase
Craving Control: Fasting can help regulate blood sugar levels, potentially helping manage cravings that are common during this phase.
Mood Stabilization: While fluctuations in mood are common during the

luteal phase, fasting might assist in balancing mood through the regulation of certain neurotransmitters.

Enhanced Digestion: Some women experience bloating or digestive discomfort in the lead-up to menstruation. Fasting can support optimal gut function, potentially alleviating some of these symptoms.

Support for Cellular Repair: Fasting promotes autophagy, a cellular cleaning process, which can be beneficial during this preparatory phase.

Fasting Strategies for the Luteal Phase

Duration: Considering the body's heightened needs, shorter fasts may be more appropriate during this phase. A 12:12 method, involving a 12-hour fast followed by a 12-hour eating window, is often suitable.

Hydration: Hydration is crucial to counteract bloating. Opt for herbal teas like chamomile or ginger, known for their soothing properties.

Nutrient Intake: Prioritize magnesium-rich foods, such as nuts, seeds, and leafy greens, to alleviate muscle cramps and mood swings. Also, consume adequate healthy fats, like avocados and olive oil, as progesterone production relies on cholesterol.

Manage Stress: Engage in relaxation techniques like deep breathing or light stretching. It can help manage mood swings and PMS symptoms.

Confronting Challenges in the Luteal Phase

1. **Pronounced Cravings:** It's natural for many to crave sweets or salty foods. Instead of resisting, opt for healthier versions, like dark chocolate or roasted nuts.
2. **Fatigue:** Energy levels might dip during this phase. Listen to the body's signals and avoid rigorous fasting or strenuous workouts.
3. **Emotional Swings:** Hormonal changes can affect mood. It's essential to prioritize self-care, possibly integrating mindfulness or journaling practices.

The luteal phase encapsulates the body's incredible capacity for creation and renewal. Embracing its rhythms and supporting the body's needs through tailored fasting can make the transition to the menstrual phase smoother and more harmonious.

As the menstrual cycle comes full circle, it brings along lessons of adaptability, resilience, and the marvel that is the female body. The next phase is the return to menstruation, marking both an end and a beginning. Understanding this cycle and adapting fasting practices provides a pathway to empowerment, allowing every woman to harness her unique strength, irrespective of the phase she's navigating.

Intermittent fasting and cycle syncing: A weekly plan

Intermittent fasting and cycle syncing have emerged as powerful tools for women looking to optimize their health, energy, and well-being. By understanding the unique hormonal landscape of each menstrual phase, women can tailor their fasting approach to align with their body's needs, creating a synergy that amplifies benefits and reduces potential challenges.

The Power of Syncing Fasting with the Menstrual Cycle

Integrating intermittent fasting with the body's natural rhythms can lead to:

Enhanced Energy Levels: Tailored fasting can optimize energy utilization throughout the menstrual cycle.

Balanced Moods: By aligning fasting windows with hormonal shifts, mood swings can be better managed.

Optimal Digestion: Fasting strategies can alleviate some digestive discomforts experienced during different phases.

Empowerment: Women can feel more in tune with their bodies, taking charge of their health and well-being.

A Weekly Plan for Intermittent Fasting and Cycle Syncing

Week 1 - Menstrual Phase (Days 1-7): Gentle Fasting

Fasting Duration: Opt for shorter fasting windows, such as 10:14 or 12:12.

Focus Foods: Iron-rich foods like spinach, legumes, and red meat can be beneficial due to menstrual blood loss. Also, integrate hydrating foods like cucumbers and watermelon.

Activity Level: Opt for light activities like walking or gentle yoga to support circulation and alleviate cramps.

Week 2 - Follicular Phase (Days 8-13): Fueling Fertility

Fasting Duration: As energy levels rise, fasting windows can be extended. A 14:10 or 16:8 approach can be adopted.

Focus Foods: Zinc-rich foods, such as pumpkin seeds, cashews, and chickpeas, can support egg development. Fresh fruits and vegetables can enhance overall vitality.

Activity Level: Engage in moderate to high-intensity workouts, reflecting the body's increasing energy.

Week 3 - Ovulation Phase (Days 14-17): Balancing Act

Fasting Duration: With heightened insulin sensitivity, a 14:10 method can strike the right balance.

Focus Foods: Whole grains, lean proteins, and omega-3 rich foods can stabilize blood sugar levels and support hormonal balance.

Activity Level: Continue with moderate-intensity workouts, while also incorporating flexibility exercises.

Week 4 - Luteal Phase (Days 18-28): Prepping for the Fast

Fasting Duration: Shorter fasts, like 12:12, can align with the body's heightened needs.

Focus Foods: Magnesium-rich foods can alleviate muscle cramps and mood swings. Prioritize healthy fats to support progesterone production.

Activity Level: Opt for low to moderate-intensity workouts, with a focus on relaxation and stress management.

Navigating the Fasting and Syncing Journey

1. **Listen to the Body:** The above plan is a guideline. Individual needs

may vary, so it's essential to tune into the body's signals.

2. **Stay Hydrated:** Regardless of the phase, hydration is crucial. It supports detoxification, aids digestion, and can alleviate various symptoms.

3. **Adapt and Evolve:** Over time, the body's response to fasting may change. Regularly assess how fasting feels during different phases and adjust accordingly.

4. **Seek Support:** Engaging in a community or seeking guidance from experts can provide additional insights and motivation.

5. **Celebrate Small Wins:** Recognize the progress made. Whether it's improved energy, better mood balance, or heightened awareness, every step forward counts.

The concept of intermittent fasting and cycle syncing represents a holistic approach to health and well-being. By aligning fasting practices with the menstrual cycle, women can harness the innate wisdom of their bodies, paving the way for enhanced vitality, balance, and empowerment. This journey underscores the profound interconnectedness of systems within the body and illuminates the path to holistic health.

5

Fasting Protocols and Fat Burning

Intermittent Fasting: A path to fat loss

Intermittent fasting has captured global attention for its transformative effects on health, longevity, and weight management. Central to these benefits is its potent impact on fat loss. By manipulating the body's metabolic machinery, intermittent fasting taps into stored fat reserves, promoting efficient weight loss while retaining muscle mass.

The Metabolic Magic Behind Intermittent Fasting

The body primarily runs on glucose, a type of sugar sourced from daily food intake. In the absence of this immediate fuel source, as is the case during fasting, the body looks for alternatives. This shift leads to the mobilization of stored fat for energy. The liver breaks down these fat reserves, producing molecules called ketones, which serve as a potent fuel source for the brain and body.

Benefits of Targeted Fat Loss Through Fasting

Visceral Fat Reduction: Intermittent fasting particularly targets visceral fat, a type of fat stored in the abdomen. Excessive visceral fat is linked to numerous health risks, including cardiovascular diseases and insulin resistance.

Preservation of Muscle Mass: Unlike many other weight loss strategies that can lead to muscle degradation, intermittent fasting promotes fat loss while largely retaining lean muscle tissue.

Boosted Metabolism: Contrary to the belief that fasting might slow down metabolism, short-term fasting can actually boost metabolic rate, promoting faster calorie burn.

Enhanced Brain Health: The ketones produced from fat breakdown have neuroprotective properties, supporting cognitive function and reducing the risk of neurodegenerative diseases.

Popular Intermittent Fasting Protocols for Fat Loss

16/8 Method: Involves fasting for 16 hours a day and eating all meals within an 8-hour window. This pattern can be repeated daily or several times a week.

24-hour Fasts: This entails fasting from dinner one day to dinner the next day, translating to a full 24-hour fast. It can be done once or twice a week.

5:2 Diet: Involves consuming regular diet five days a week, followed by two days of restricted calorie intake, usually capped at 500-600 calories.

Alternate Day Fasting: As the name suggests, followers eat normally one day and fast or consume very few calories the next.

Warrior Diet: This protocol consists of fasting for 20 hours and eating one large meal in the evening.

Tips for Optimizing Fat Loss During Fasting

Stay Hydrated: Drinking ample water supports metabolism and can help curb hunger pangs.

Prioritize Protein: When breaking the fast, focus on protein-rich foods. Protein supports muscle maintenance and growth, and its digestion burns more calories than the digestion of fats or carbohydrates.

Integrate Strength Training: Incorporate resistance training exercises.

This can help maintain or even build muscle mass during fasting, further enhancing metabolic rate.

Limit Added Sugars: Sugary foods and drinks can cause blood sugar spikes, potentially hampering fat loss. Opt for whole, unprocessed foods.

Rest and Recover: Sleep plays a pivotal role in weight management. Ensure 7-9 hours of quality sleep each night to support fat loss and overall health.

Addressing Concerns Around Fasting and Fat Loss

1. **Hunger Pangs:** Initially, feelings of hunger might be pronounced. Over time, as the body adjusts, these sensations often diminish.
2. **Potential Nutrient Deficiencies:** Extended or frequent fasting without mindful eating during eating windows can lead to nutrient deficiencies. It's vital to focus on nutrient-dense foods and consider supplementation if needed.
3. **Overeating Post-Fast:** Some might feel the urge to overcompensate for the fasting period by eating excessively. Structured meal planning can counteract this tendency.

Intermittent fasting, when practiced mindfully, offers a sustainable approach to fat loss. It shifts the body's metabolic focus, prioritizes stored fat as a primary energy source, and promotes weight loss without compromising muscle mass. Understanding the principles behind this practice and integrating complementary strategies ensures maximum benefits. By harnessing the metabolic power of intermittent fasting, individuals embark on a journey to a leaner, healthier self, reflecting the true essence of freedom in health.

Extended Fasts: Benefits and Precautions

Beyond the popular intermittent fasting methods lies the realm of extended fasting. This approach often involves abstaining from food for periods exceeding 48 hours. While the concept may seem daunting, extended fasting offers a unique set of benefits, distinct from its shorter-duration counterparts. However, understanding its potential advantages and precautions is crucial for anyone considering this profound metabolic experience.

Deep Dive into Extended Fasting

Extended fasting catapults the body into a more profound metabolic switch. Beyond the primary stages of glucose depletion, the body starts to rely heavily on ketones. This reliance on fat stores rather than immediate glucose sources deepens the fat-burning effects.

The Multifaceted Benefits of Extended Fasts

Autophagy Activation: Autophagy is the body's cellular "clean-up" mechanism. During extended fasts, autophagy is activated more robustly, leading to the removal of damaged cells and the regeneration of newer, healthier ones.

Greater Insulin Sensitivity: Extended periods without food intake can enhance insulin sensitivity, potentially benefiting those with type 2 diabetes or at risk for the condition.

Heightened Mental Clarity: Many practitioners report a heightened sense of clarity and focus during extended fasts, attributed to the brain's use of ketones as a primary fuel source.

Reduction in Inflammation: Extended fasting may help reduce markers of inflammation in the body, providing benefits for a myriad of health conditions rooted in inflammatory processes.

Enhanced Growth Hormone Production: Growth hormone aids in muscle preservation and growth. Extended fasting can lead to spikes in this hormone, offering potential anti-aging benefits and muscle maintenance.

Cautionary Tales: Precautions to Heed

While the benefits of extended fasting can be tantalizing, it's essential to approach with caution and awareness.

Electrolyte Imbalance: Extended fasting can lead to an imbalance in vital electrolytes. Supplementing with sodium, potassium, and magnesium can be crucial.

Refeeding Syndrome: A rare but serious risk involves refeeding syndrome, where reintroducing food too rapidly post-fast leads to a dangerous shift in fluids and electrolytes.

Potential Muscle Loss: While intermittent fasting is known to preserve muscle, extended fasting without appropriate precautions might lead to muscle degradation.

Mental Health Effects: Extended fasts can sometimes trigger or exacerbate underlying mental health conditions like anxiety or disordered eating patterns.

Medical Conditions and Medications: Those with specific medical conditions or on certain medications should consult with a healthcare professional before embarking on an extended fast.

Guidelines for a Safe Extended Fast

Stay Hydrated: Water intake remains crucial. While it's essential not to overhydrate, ensuring adequate water consumption supports detoxification and metabolic processes.

Prioritize Electrolytes: As mentioned, sodium, potassium, and magnesium are vital. Consider bone broth or electrolyte supplements.

Break the Fast Gently: When ending an extended fast, start with easily digestible foods. Bone broth, steamed vegetables, or small portions of lean protein can be ideal.

Listen to the Body: The body offers signals. If feelings of extreme discomfort, dizziness, or other adverse effects arise, it's essential to listen and potentially break the fast.

Seek Guidance: Especially for those new to extended fasting, seeking guidance from experts or experienced practitioners can offer additional insights and safety nets.

Extended fasting represents a deeper dive into the body's metabolic reservoirs. While it promises profound benefits, from enhanced cellular cleanup to heightened mental clarity, it also demands respect and caution. By understanding the potential advantages and pitfalls, and by equipping oneself with knowledge and precautions, extended fasting can be integrated safely into one's health journey. This journey, though challenging, offers transformative potential, echoing the essence of genuine freedom in well-being.

Fasting-mimicking diets: A softer approach

For many, the idea of completely abstaining from food for extended periods can be intimidating or even medically inadvisable. Here lies the beauty of fasting-mimicking diets (FMD). These diets emulate the benefits of traditional fasting while allowing for limited caloric intake. Designed to trick the body into entering a fasting state, FMDs offer a gentler approach, making the advantages of fasting more accessible to a broader audience.

Understanding the Fasting-Mimicking Paradigm

A fasting-mimicking diet typically consists of a reduced calorie intake spread over several days, often ranging from 3 to 5 days. The caloric content is carefully structured: low in proteins and sugars, and high in healthy fats. This composition nudges the body into a pseudo-fasting mode, promoting similar cellular and metabolic changes as seen in actual fasting scenarios.

Advantages of Embracing Fasting-Mimicking Diets

Cellular Regeneration: Just like traditional fasting, FMD promotes autophagy. The body clears out old, malfunctioning cells, paving the way for the generation of new, functional ones.

Reduced Risk Factors for Ageing and Diseases: Initial research indicates that FMD can decrease risk factors related to aging, diabetes, cardiovascular diseases, and some cancers.

Enhanced Cognitive Function: Beneficial changes in brain structure and cognitive function, stemming from neuroprotective properties, are seen in FMD, akin to prolonged fasting.

Fat Loss Without Muscle Wastage: The body taps into fat reserves for energy during FMD, similar to extended fasting, but the limited protein intake prevents significant muscle loss.

Improved Gut Health: With a carefully chosen caloric intake, FMD can positively influence gut health, enhancing the gut microbiome's diversity and function.

Practical Implementation of Fasting-Mimicking Diets

Caloric Breakdown: Typically, the first day of FMD consists of 1,100 calories (10% protein, 56% fat, 34% carbs), followed by around 800 calories (9% protein, 44% fat, 47% carbs) on subsequent days.

Food Choices: Opt for plant-based foods. Include nuts for healthy fats, complex carbs from vegetables, and a small amount of plant protein. Avoid animal products, high-glycemic index foods, and excessive protein.

Duration: Most FMDs last between 3 to 5 days, after which a regular, healthy diet is resumed.

Frequency: Depending on individual goals, FMD can be adopted once a month or every other month.

Safety and Considerations for Fasting-Mimicking Diets

Not for Everyone: Pregnant or breastfeeding women, individuals with a history of eating disorders, or those underweight should avoid FMD.

Monitor Blood Sugar: Those with diabetes or blood sugar issues should regularly monitor levels and consult with a healthcare professional before and during FMD.

Possible Side Effects: Just as with any fasting protocol, some may experience fatigue, dizziness, headaches, or irritability during FMD.

Post-Diet Transition: After completing an FMD, gradually reintroduce a regular diet. Start with easily digestible foods and increase caloric intake progressively.

The fasting-mimicking diet offers a bridge, a middle ground between rigorous fasting protocols and regular eating patterns. It captures the essence of fasting benefits without pushing one's boundaries excessively. In this softer approach lies an invitation: an opportunity for individuals to explore the world of fasting benefits, even if they aren't ready or able to dive into prolonged fasting. It reaffirms the notion that the path to health and freedom offers multiple routes, each adaptable and valuable in its own right.

Fat Loss vs. Weight Loss: Understanding the Difference

In the realm of health and fitness, the terms "fat loss" and "weight loss" are frequently used interchangeably. Yet, while they may sound synonymous, the underlying processes and implications differ significantly. Differentiating between these two concepts is pivotal for anyone looking to optimize their health, achieve specific fitness goals, and understand the genuine impact of fasting protocols.

Defining the Terms

Weight Loss: A decrease in total body mass, encompassing not just fat, but also water, muscle, bone, and other bodily components. Weight loss is what most standard scales reflect, offering a holistic view of one's body composition changes but not detailing the specifics.

Fat Loss: A reduction in body fat, both the visible fat located beneath the skin (subcutaneous) and the deeper, visceral fat surrounding internal organs. Fat loss zeroes in on the body's adipose tissue, targeting the stored lipids without necessarily impacting other body components as directly.

Why the Distinction Matters

Health Implications: Losing weight doesn't always equate to improved health. For instance, rapid weight loss can sometimes involve muscle wastage, leading to decreased strength and potential metabolic slowdowns. Fat loss, especially when visceral fat is reduced, typically carries more direct health benefits.

Aesthetic Outcomes: Many individuals chase a toned, defined physique. Achieving this look necessitates fat loss rather than just weight loss. One could lose weight, but if it's primarily from muscle, the desired aesthetic might remain elusive.

Metabolic Considerations: Muscle tissue is metabolically active, meaning it burns calories even at rest. If weight loss involves significant muscle depletion, one's resting metabolic rate (the energy expended while at rest) could decrease, potentially making future fat loss more challenging.

Fitness Goals: Athletes and fitness enthusiasts often need to maintain or build muscle while shedding fat. Understanding the difference between fat and weight loss ensures they can tailor their nutrition and exercise regimens accordingly.

Navigating Weight and Fat Loss During Fasting

Fasting protocols, especially when combined with specific exercise routines, can be geared towards promoting fat loss while preserving muscle.

Intermittent Fasting: By cycling between eating and fasting windows, intermittent fasting can promote fat loss, especially when combined with resistance training, which aids muscle preservation.

Extended Fasting: While extended fasting primarily targets fat reserves for energy, prolonged periods without protein intake might risk muscle loss. Hence, such fasts should be approached with caution, ensuring adequate protein intake upon breaking the fast.

Fasting-Mimicking Diets: As previously explored, these diets promote fat loss without significantly impacting muscle mass, providing a balanced approach.

Measuring Fat Loss Over Weight Loss

Body Composition Scans: Devices like DEXA scans or bioelectrical impedance scales provide detailed insights into one's fat percentage, muscle mass, and bone density.

Measurements: Using a tape measure to track changes in waist, hip, and other body parts can indicate fat loss, especially if measurements decrease while strength levels remain consistent.

Photos: Regular progress photos can visually capture changes in body composition over time.

Functional Indicators: Strength levels, endurance, and how one's clothes fit can also offer cues about changes in fat vs. muscle.

The journey towards optimal health and desired aesthetics isn't merely a game of numbers. It's about understanding what those numbers represent and how they interplay with one's unique body and goals. In the dance of fat and weight loss, knowledge empowers individuals to make informed decisions, ensuring that their chosen path aligns with their health aspirations and desired outcomes. With fasting protocols as tools, the possibility to sculpt, redefine, and rejuvenate the body becomes a tangible reality, echoing once more the core message of freedom in well-being.

Combining Fasting Protocols for Optimal Fat Burning

Harnessing the power of multiple fasting protocols can provide a potent tool in the quest for fat loss. By understanding each protocol's strengths and potential synergies, it's possible to create a tailored, dynamic approach to optimizing fat burning while ensuring overall health and vitality.

The Power of Combining

Drawing upon the strengths of various fasting methods can yield benefits that outstrip those achieved through any single protocol. A combination can:

Prevent Plateaus: The body is adept at adapting. Over time, relying on one fasting protocol might yield diminishing returns. Rotation can keep the body responsive.

Provide Nutritional Balance: Extended fasting, while powerful, can lead to nutrient deficiencies if practiced continuously. Interspersing it with milder fasting protocols or fasting-mimicking diets can ensure adequate nutrient intake.

Optimize Hormonal Response: Different fasting methods trigger diverse hormonal reactions. For instance, while short-term fasts boost growth hormone production, longer fasts might enhance insulin sensitivity. A combined approach can offer a balanced hormonal environment conducive to fat loss.

Strategies for Combining Fasting Protocols

Intermittent Fasting as a Foundation: Given its flexible nature, intermittent fasting (IF) can serve as a foundational practice. One might choose a daily 16:8 protocol (16 hours of fasting followed by an 8-hour eating window).

Incorporating Extended Fasts: Once accustomed to IF, an occasional extended fast, perhaps once a month or once every two months, can amplify fat-burning processes. These fasts, lasting anywhere from 48 hours to a week, can act as a metabolic reset.

Using Fasting-Mimicking Diets for Transition: After an extended fast, transitioning with a fasting-mimicking diet can provide the body with a gentle reintroduction to regular caloric intake, ensuring that the benefits of the extended fast are consolidated while restoring nutrient balance.

Cyclical Approaches: One might also consider a cyclical approach, such as two weeks of intermittent fasting followed by a 5-day fasting-mimicking diet. This cycle can then be repeated, interspersed with occasional extended fasts.

Exercise Integration for Enhanced Fat Burning

Strength Training: Especially crucial during intermittent fasting windows, strength training can help preserve muscle mass, ensuring that weight loss primarily targets fat.

Low-Intensity Steady-State (LISS) Cardio: During fasting windows, especially in the morning, LISS cardio (like walking or leisurely cycling) can optimize fat utilization for energy.

High-Intensity Interval Training (HIIT): Best practiced during eating windows, HIIT can enhance metabolic rate and stimulate growth hormone production, further bolstering fat loss.

Mindful Monitoring and Customization

As with any regimen, monitoring one's response is crucial:

Biofeedback: Regularly check in with one's energy levels, mood, sleep quality, and hunger sensations. These can offer cues about how the body is responding and whether adjustments are needed.

Objective Measures: Utilize body composition scans, measurements, and weight tracking to gauge progress. However, remember that day-to-day fluctuations are natural.

Adjust Based on Life's Demands: During particularly stressful times or periods of high physical demand, it might be advisable to ease up on rigorous fasting protocols. Listen to the body and adapt.

Consultation: Especially when combining multiple fasting methods, consulting with healthcare or nutrition professionals can provide valuable insights and safety checks.

The tapestry of fasting is rich and varied. When individual threads — each representing a unique protocol — are woven together, the result is a powerful fabric capable of supporting optimal fat loss and holistic health. This integrative approach showcases fasting's versatility, ensuring that each person can find or craft a path that resonates with their goals, lifestyle, and well-being aspirations. It's a testament to the adaptability and resilience of the human body, and the myriad ways in which we can nurture, challenge, and rejuvenate it.

6

Overcoming Common Fasting Challenges

Overcoming hunger and cravings

Hunger, an age-old companion of mankind, has been the driving force behind many of our evolutionary adaptations. It has led us to hunt, to gather, to innovate, and to find new ways to sustain ourselves. But in the modern age of abundance, hunger plays a different role in our lives, especially when one is committed to the fasting journey.

Fasting, as beneficial as it may be, isn't devoid of challenges. One of the primary hurdles encountered is the potent sensation of hunger and the food cravings that tag along. These can sometimes make fasting particularly demanding. Especially for women, with the unique ebb and flow of hormones that might intensify these feelings, understanding hunger and finding strategies to manage it is paramount.

Understanding the Science Behind Hunger

Before diving into the management techniques, it's essential to understand what happens in our bodies when we feel hungry. Hunger is not just a monolithic sensation; it's a nuanced interplay of hormones, primarily ghrelin - often labeled the "hunger hormone". When the stomach is empty, ghrelin is produced. Upon eating, ghrelin levels drop. It's a signal, essentially, that communicates between the stomach and the brain, particularly the hypothalamus.

For women, the interplay is even more intricate. The menstrual cycle influences ghrelin levels. Typically, during the luteal phase, the post-ovulation period leading up to menstruation, women might experience heightened hunger and cravings. This is nature's way of potentially preparing the body for a possible pregnancy.

Differentiating Between Hunger and Appetite

It's crucial to understand that hunger and appetite are not synonyms. Hunger is the physiological need for food - the body signaling that it requires nourishment. Appetite, on the other hand, is a psychological desire to eat. It's not about needing food but wanting it. This distinction is vital in a fasting journey, as recognizing true hunger from a fleeting appetite can make all the difference.

Strategies to Overcome Hunger and Cravings

Stay Hydrated: Many times, our bodies confuse thirst with hunger. Drinking ample water can keep hunger at bay and help in detoxification during fasting.

Balanced Diet: When not fasting, ensure you're eating a balanced diet. Nutrient deficiencies can lead to increased hunger and cravings. For women, ensuring a good intake of iron, magnesium, and Vitamin B6 can help, especially during the menstrual cycle.

Mindful Eating: Paying attention to what you eat, savoring each bite, and being present during meals can reduce the amount you eat and improve satisfaction, helping to curb hunger later.

Distraction: When a craving strikes, divert your attention. Take a walk, read a book, or engage in an activity. Often, the craving will pass.

Sleep Well: Lack of sleep can increase ghrelin production. Ensure you're getting quality sleep every night.

Herbal Teas: Warm beverages can provide a feeling of fullness. Herbal teas, in particular, can be soothing and can often help curb appetite.

Understand Your Triggers: Are you truly hungry, or is it an emotional response? Identifying patterns can be crucial. If you tend to eat when you're stressed or anxious, finding alternative coping mechanisms can be beneficial.

Supplements: Some supplements might help manage hunger. However, always consult with a healthcare professional before incorporating any new supplements.

Reassess Your Fasting Window: Remember, fasting is not one-size-fits-all. If you're struggling too much, it might be worth reassessing your fasting windows or trying different fasting methods.

Positive Affirmations: The mind is a powerful tool. Remind yourself of the reasons you're on this fasting journey, the health benefits, and the empowerment it brings.

Cravings, Hormones, and Embracing the Journey

It's also vital to remember that cravings, especially for women, can be hormonally driven. As mentioned earlier, the luteal phase can be a particularly challenging time. But understanding this can arm you with the tools and the mindset to navigate these challenges. Maybe it means being gentler on yourself during these periods or finding specific strategies that work best for you.

In the grand tapestry of your fasting journey, these moments of hunger, of craving, are but threads weaving the larger picture. Embrace them, understand them, and know that every challenge is an opportunity for growth. Remember, the fasting journey is not just about the destination, but the lessons and empowerment acquired along the way.

Tackling Emotional and Stress Eating

Modern life often throws emotional and mental challenges at us, leading many to find solace in food. For millennia, food has been more than just sustenance; it has been comfort, celebration, and even an act of love. This cultural and emotional connection to food can make the fasting journey complex, especially when encountering stress or overwhelming emotions.

Unraveling the Roots of Emotional Eating

Emotional eating refers to the consumption of food for reasons other than hunger. An individual might turn to food to cope with stress, sadness, anxiety, boredom, or even joy. This form of eating does not arise from a physical need to eat but from an emotional desire.

Stress eating, a subset of emotional eating, specifically involves consuming food in response to stressors. When stressed, the body produces a hormone called cortisol. Elevated cortisol levels can lead to increased appetite, especially for sugary, fatty, or salty foods.

For women, the relationship with food and emotions can be further complicated by hormonal fluctuations throughout the menstrual cycle, which can amplify feelings and reactions. Recognizing these patterns is the first step in tackling emotional and stress eating.

Identifying Emotional Eating Triggers

Personal Triggers: Emotional eaters need to recognize what events, places, or feelings trigger their desire to eat. It could be as straightforward as specific dates on the calendar or as complex as certain emotional states.

Physical Sensations: Paying attention to physical sensations can help differentiate between actual hunger and emotional hunger. Emotional hunger usually appears suddenly, demanding instant satisfaction, while genuine hunger arises gradually.

Food Choices: Emotional eaters often crave junk food or comfort food. Identifying these specific foods can be a clear sign of emotional eating.

Mindless Eating: If you find yourself eating without paying attention to the act, it's a significant indicator of emotional eating.

After-Eating Feelings: True hunger satisfaction leaves one feeling energized. In contrast, emotional eating often leads to feelings of guilt or regret.

Techniques to Counter Emotional and Stress Eating

Mindfulness and Meditation: Engaging in mindfulness practices can create awareness about eating habits. Meditation can serve as a tool to manage stress, reducing the inclination to resort to food for comfort.

Balanced Diet: Keeping a balanced diet ensures that the body is well-nourished and reduces cravings. A deficiency in essential nutrients can sometimes manifest as cravings for specific foods.

Healthy Alternatives: Replace unhealthy snacks with nutritious alternatives. When the urge to eat strikes, having a healthy option can make a big difference.

Physical Activity: Engaging in physical activities can serve as a distraction and help release pent-up emotions. It's also a great way to reduce stress.

Talk About It: Sometimes, just talking to someone about what you're feeling can help process emotions. Sharing with a friend or a support group can be therapeutic.

Limit Exposure to Stressors: If specific situations or people tend to stress you out, try to limit your exposure to them or find coping mechanisms to handle those situations better.

Professional Help: If emotional or stress eating becomes a chronic issue, it might be beneficial to seek help from a therapist or counselor who specializes in eating disorders.

Journaling: Keeping a journal can be an effective way to recognize patterns in emotional eating. Writing down what you eat, when you eat, and most importantly, how you felt when you ate can provide valuable insights.

Pause Before Eating: When the urge to eat strikes, take a moment to ask yourself why you want to eat. Is it genuine hunger? Or is it an emotion driving you? Sometimes, just pausing can create a significant shift.

Environment Matters: Create an environment that doesn't support emotional eating. This might mean not stocking up on unhealthy snacks or even creating a designated eating area where you eat mindfully.

Coping with Hormonal Fluctuations and Emotional Eating

For many women, hormonal fluctuations throughout the menstrual cycle can intensify emotional responses. Recognizing that hormones can exacerbate emotional eating tendencies can help in creating strategies specific to different phases of the cycle. For instance, during the luteal phase, when emotional eating tendencies might be heightened, practicing extra mindfulness or engaging in activities that help in emotion regulation can be beneficial.

Emotional and stress eating is a complex issue intertwined with our biology, environment, past experiences, and individual personalities. While fasting presents an additional layer of challenge, understanding the nuances of one's relationship with food and emotions can pave the way for a harmonious fasting journey. Remember, fasting is not just about abstaining from food but about building a healthier relationship with it. Every challenge faced and overcome reinforces the strength and resilience inherent in every woman.

Busting through Fat Loss Plateaus

Every fasting and weight loss journey comes with its unique challenges. One such challenge that many women face, regardless of their fasting protocol, is the dreaded fat loss plateau. After weeks or even months of consistent weight and fat loss, suddenly the scale doesn't budge. Despite best efforts and strict adherence to the fasting regimen, fat loss seems to have come to a standstill.

Understanding what a plateau is, why it occurs, and strategies to overcome it are crucial for those committed to achieving and maintaining their fat loss goals.

Defining a Fat Loss Plateau

A fat loss plateau occurs when there is no change in body weight for an extended period, typically two weeks or longer. It's important to differentiate between weight loss and fat loss. Weight can fluctuate daily due to factors like water retention, muscle gain, or digestive contents, but a true fat loss plateau signifies that the body is not burning excess fat despite maintaining a caloric deficit.

Reasons Behind a Fat Loss Plateau

Adaptive Thermogenesis: As one loses weight, the body requires fewer calories to function. It adapts to this new normal by slowing down metabolic processes, a phenomenon termed adaptive thermogenesis.

Loss of Lean Muscle Mass: Muscle is metabolically active, meaning it burns calories even at rest. If muscle mass decreases, so does the basal metabolic rate, making it harder to maintain a caloric deficit.

Hormonal Changes: Extended periods of caloric restriction can impact hormones that regulate appetite and metabolism, like leptin and ghrelin.

Decreased Activity: As one loses weight, there's less body mass to move around, leading to fewer calories burned through daily activities.

Overestimation of Caloric Burn: It's common to overestimate the number of calories burned through exercise and underestimate the calories consumed.

Strategies to Break Through the Plateau

Reassess Caloric Intake: As one's weight drops, caloric needs change. It might be time to adjust daily caloric intake to match the new metabolic rate.

Switch Up the Fasting Routine: If one has been following a 16:8 intermittent fasting routine, it might help to try a 20:4 routine or even a 24-hour fast. Changing the pattern can sometimes jolt the body out of its plateau.

Increase Protein Intake: Protein can boost metabolism for a few hours by inducing the thermic effect of food, which is the energy required to digest, absorb, and process nutrients. Additionally, protein can help preserve lean muscle mass.

Strength Training: Incorporating or increasing strength training can help build or maintain muscle mass, thus boosting the metabolic rate.

High-Intensity Interval Training (HIIT): This form of exercise can increase metabolic rate for hours after the workout is completed.

Stay Hydrated: Drinking enough water can help with fat metabolism and reduce the chances of mistaking thirst for hunger.

Get Quality Sleep: Poor sleep can affect hormones that regulate appetite and fat storage.

Practice Stress Management: Chronic stress can lead to hormonal imbalances that promote fat storage.

Consider a Diet Break: Taking a short break from caloric restriction, while still eating mindfully, can sometimes reset some of the hormonal changes caused by prolonged deficits.

Keep a Food Diary: Tracking food can provide insights into any unintentional overeating or patterns that could be hindering fat loss.

Be Patient and Trust the Process: Bodies are complex, and sometimes they need time to adjust. Stay consistent, and remember that plateaus are a natural part of any weight loss journey.

Hormonal Considerations for Women

For women, especially those in the reproductive age, hormonal fluctuations across the menstrual cycle can affect weight and fat loss. For example, during the luteal phase, women may experience increased appetite and water retention, which can mask fat loss on the scale. Being aware of these hormonal changes and adjusting expectations and strategies accordingly can be beneficial.

Additionally, women approaching menopause or in menopause might face challenges due to decreased estrogen levels, which can lead to a lower metabolic rate. In such cases, a combination of dietary adjustments, strength training, and hormone therapy (if advised by a healthcare provider) can be effective.

Remember the Non-Scale Victories

While breaking through a fat loss plateau is a goal, it's essential to remember the other benefits of fasting and healthy lifestyle choices. Improved energy levels, better mental clarity, enhanced mood, and overall well-being are just as vital, if not more so, than the number on the scale.

Challenges, including plateaus, are inevitable in any journey. They test resolve, patience, and adaptability. By understanding the body, especially the unique challenges women face, and by arming oneself with knowledge and strategies, it becomes possible to overcome these plateaus and continue on the path to optimal health and well-being.

Addressing Social Pressures and Maintaining a Social Life

The societal tapestry is intricately woven with threads of food, celebration, and community. From Sunday brunches to festive feasts, our social lives often revolve around meals. When fasting becomes a significant part of one's routine, the question naturally arises: How does one navigate the social landscape without jeopardizing relationships or the benefits of fasting?

Navigating this new terrain can feel like walking a tightrope, but with understanding, planning, and a bit of creativity, one can confidently maintain both fasting commitments and a vibrant social life.

Understanding the Roots of Social Pressures

Our relationship with food is deeply embedded in cultural, familial, and social norms. Generations have passed down rituals that involve communal meals, shared dishes, and gastronomic celebrations. Against this backdrop, choosing not to partake in eating when everyone else is can invite questions, concerns, or even critiques.

Respecting Tradition While Honoring Personal Choices

Maintaining respect for traditions and social norms is crucial. However, honoring personal health choices is equally vital. To strike this balance:

Plan Ahead: If invited to a dinner, consider adjusting fasting hours to allow participation in the meal. Alternatively, if a fasting window cannot be shifted, attend the gathering and enjoy non-caloric beverages.

Communicate: Being open about fasting choices helps in setting expectations. Share reasons for fasting, focusing on health and personal benefits rather than weight loss alone.

Be Prepared for Questions: Curiosity will arise. Arm oneself with knowledge about fasting's benefits, and answer queries with confidence. Remember, it's okay to keep explanations simple and steer the conversation away if it becomes uncomfortable.

Offer to Host: By hosting gatherings, control over the menu and timing remains in one's hands. It provides an opportunity to introduce friends and family to fasting-friendly meals.

Focus on Non-Food Activities: Socializing doesn't always have to center around meals. Propose activities like movie nights, hikes, or museum visits.

Overcoming the Fear of Missing Out (FOMO)

It's natural to feel like one is missing out on delicious dishes or festive feasts. However, reframing the perspective can be powerful. Instead of focusing on what is being missed, concentrate on the gains from fasting: enhanced energy, improved health markers, mental clarity, and the joy of achieving personal health goals.

Dealing with Peer Pressure and Unwanted Opinions

Fasting might not be the norm in many social circles. Thus, decisions to fast may be met with skepticism, concern, or even mild ridicule. Here's how to handle such situations:

Stay Confident: Remember the reasons for embarking on the fasting journey. Personal health and well-being are paramount.

Seek Support: Connect with like-minded individuals or communities that understand and support fasting. Sharing experiences and challenges with those on a similar journey can be immensely comforting.

Educate Tactfully: When met with concern or skepticism, gently share information about the benefits and safety of fasting. Sometimes, resistance stems from misinformation or lack of knowledge.

Set Boundaries: It's okay to assertively but politely decline food offers or change the topic if discussions about fasting become intrusive or negative.

The Balancing Act: Social Life and Fasting

Remember, fasting is flexible. If a special occasion arises, it's okay to adjust fasting windows or take a break. Life is to be enjoyed, and fostering connections with loved ones is essential.

Being Present

In social settings, even if not partaking in meals, one can be wholly present. Engage in conversations, listen actively, and enjoy the company of loved ones. Often, it's the shared laughter, stories, and experiences that linger in memory, not the meals.

Practicing Self-Compassion

Every fasting journey will have its unique challenges, including navigating the social landscape. Mistakes, misjudgments, or moments of weakness might occur. Instead of self-criticism, practice self-compassion. Understand that the journey is a marathon, not a sprint, and every step, even the missteps, is part of the learning process.

In the dance of fasting and socializing, there will be moments of grace and moments of stumble. But with understanding, planning, and a sprinkle of creativity, it is entirely possible to glide seamlessly through social settings, honoring both personal health choices and the joy of shared moments.

Ensuring Nutritional Adequacy During Fasts

The essence of fasting is abstinence from food for designated periods, but this raises a valid concern. How does one ensure that they're receiving all essential nutrients when food consumption is limited or entirely absent for extended hours? The answer lies in a meticulous blend of informed food choices, supplement considerations, and understanding the body's unique requirements.

Nutritional Needs: An Overview

Each individual requires a host of macro and micronutrients to function optimally. Macronutrients are the proteins, fats, and carbohydrates that provide energy. Micronutrients, though required in tiny amounts, play vital roles. These include vitamins, minerals, and certain other compounds. Meeting these needs during non-fasting windows ensures that the body remains nourished even when food isn't being consumed.

The Symphony of Nutrients in Fasting

When not consuming food, the body does a remarkable thing: it starts using its reserves. Stored fats become a primary energy source, and this process has its set of benefits. However, using these reserves doesn't provide all the essential nutrients, and that's where the challenge lies.

Optimizing Nutrient Intake During Eating Windows

Ensuring nutrient intake begins when the fasting window ends. Here's how to do it:

Prioritize Protein: Proteins are building blocks. Choose high-quality sources like lean meats, fish, eggs, legumes, and dairy. For vegetarians or vegans, combining different plant sources can ensure a complete amino acid profile.

Fats are Friends: Not all fats are created equal. Embrace healthy sources such as avocados, nuts, seeds, olives, and certain oils like coconut and olive. These provide essential fatty acids and are pivotal for the absorption of fat-soluble vitamins: A, D, E, and K.

Choose Complex Carbohydrates: Rather than simple sugars, opt for complex carbs found in whole grains, fruits, and vegetables. They are rich in fiber, aiding digestion and providing sustained energy.

Micronutrient Magic: Colorful vegetables and fruits, nuts, seeds, and animal products are micronutrient goldmines. Rotating through a variety of these ensures a broad spectrum of vitamins and minerals.

Hydration: While water is essential, remember that hydration isn't just about quenching thirst. Electrolytes (sodium, potassium, magnesium, and calcium) balance is crucial, especially during extended fasts. Consider bone broths, electrolyte solutions, or specific supplements if needed.

Limit Empty-Calorie Foods: Processed foods, sugary drinks, or excessive desserts might be tempting, especially after a fast. However, they provide minimal nutritional value and can interfere with the objective of nutrient optimization.

Supplementation: A Helping Hand

In certain situations, achieving nutritional adequacy through food alone becomes challenging. Here's where supplements can be beneficial:

Multivitamins: These can be an insurance policy, filling in any gaps in nutrient intake.

Minerals: Extended fasting or specific diets might lead to deficiencies in minerals like magnesium, potassium, or calcium. Supplements can help restore balance.

Vitamin D: Given its importance and the common deficiency, a Vitamin D supplement, especially in places with limited sunlight, can be considered.

Omega-3 Fatty Acids: Especially for those who don't consume fatty fish regularly, an Omega-3 supplement can be advantageous.

Special Considerations: Iron for menstruating women, B12 for vegans, or other specific supplements might be necessary based on individual circumstances.

Caution: While supplements can be beneficial, they are not a substitute for a well-rounded diet. Also, it's essential to consult with a healthcare professional before starting any supplementation regime.

Listen to the Body's Cues

The body communicates continuously. Feelings of prolonged fatigue, hair loss, brittle nails, or other unusual symptoms might signal nutritional deficiencies. Regular health check-ups, including blood tests, can shed light on any such concerns.

Planning and Preparing

Having a plan is half the battle won. Consider meal planning or even meal prepping to ensure nutrient-rich foods are readily available post fasting. Embracing this approach reduces the temptation to opt for less nutritious, convenient alternatives.

Flexibility in Fasting Regimes

If finding it challenging to meet nutritional needs within the existing fasting routine, consider adjusting the fasting protocol. Remember, the goal is overall health and well-being.

In the grand tapestry of health and well-being, fasting is a powerful tool, but like any tool, it must be used judiciously. As one navigates the fasting journey, ensuring nutritional adequacy is like setting a strong foundation upon which the magnificent edifice of health can be constructed. The choices made during eating windows lay the bricks, the body's innate wisdom acts as the architect, and the result is a resilient, nourished self, ready to embrace the challenges and joys of life.

7

Fasting and Fitness

Fasting and Muscle Preservation: Debunking Myths

In the world of fitness, muscle mass is often held in reverence, symbolizing strength, resilience, and a manifestation of dedication to physical health. Yet, when the topic of fasting surfaces in fitness circles, apprehensions arise. One prominent concern is the potential loss of hard-earned muscle. What if fasting, instead of aiding fitness goals, diminishes muscle mass? Delving deep into this subject, we'll separate facts from fiction and explore the intricate relationship between fasting and muscle preservation.

The Physiological Basis: Understanding Muscle Metabolism

Muscles aren't just for show; they play numerous roles in daily life, from moving bodies to assisting with vital functions. They store energy in the form of glycogen and amino acids. When the body is starved of external energy sources, it looks inward, and muscles seem like a potential source. But the body is smarter than given credit for. Instead of directly depleting muscles, it initiates a series of metabolic processes to source energy elsewhere, primarily from fat stores.

Fasting: Body's Primary Energy Sources

When food is abundant, carbohydrates, particularly glucose, serve as the primary energy source. During fasting, this external glucose supply dwindles. The body's first response is to utilize stored glycogen, primarily found in the liver. Once glycogen stores are exhausted, a fascinating shift occurs: the body enters ketosis, producing ketone bodies from stored fats. These ketones become the primary energy source, sparing muscles from being used as fuel.

Muscle Protein Breakdown: Not as Severe as Assumed

Yes, there's a phase where the body uses amino acids for energy, particularly in the initial stages of fasting before ketosis sets in. However, this muscle protein breakdown is not as pronounced as some assume. In fact, studies have shown that short-term fasting increases growth hormone secretion, a hormone instrumental in muscle preservation and growth.

Autophagy: Nature's Recycling Program

One of fasting's most remarkable benefits is the induction of autophagy, a cellular cleansing process. Think of it as the body's recycling program, where old, damaged proteins are broken down and used for essential functions. This not only conserves proteins but also ensures muscle health by removing potentially harmful, worn-out cellular components.

Lean Mass vs. Total Muscle Mass

It's essential to differentiate between losing muscle protein and decreasing muscle water content. Extended fasting or a shift to a ketogenic state can lead to reduced muscle glycogen and water. This might reflect as weight loss or even a slight decrease in muscle size but doesn't necessarily translate to actual muscle protein loss.

Fasting Duration Matters

Short-term fasts, like intermittent fasting, have minimal impact on muscle protein breakdown. However, very extended fasts, beyond 48 to 72 hours, might increase the risk. The key lies in finding a balance and ensuring adequate protein intake during eating windows.

Resistance Training: The Muscle Saver

While fasting has a role, preserving and even building muscle mass depends significantly on physical activity. Resistance or strength training exercises, in particular, send a strong signal to muscles. They convey a simple message: "You're essential, and we need you." This stimulation, combined with adequate protein intake post-workout, can not only preserve but also build muscle mass during fasting regimes.

Optimizing Protein Intake

Post-fast, it's not just about consuming protein, but emphasizing its quality and timing. Complete protein sources, rich in all essential amino acids, are vital. Think lean meats, dairy, eggs, or a combination of plant-based proteins like legumes and grains. Moreover, consuming protein after a workout can capitalize on the increased muscle protein synthesis that exercise offers.

Listening to Body Signals

Each body reacts differently. Some might experience muscle soreness, fatigue, or even slight muscle loss initially. Adjusting fasting durations, ensuring optimal nutrient intake, and incorporating regular resistance training can mitigate these challenges.

Muscle Preservation: A Holistic Approach

Preserving muscle mass during fasting isn't about isolating one aspect but adopting a holistic approach. From understanding body metabolism to incorporating resistance training and ensuring optimal nutrient intake, each facet intertwines to create a symphony of muscle preservation.

In this journey, it's not just about dispelling myths but embracing truths. Fasting, when approached with knowledge and a touch of intuition, can co-exist beautifully with fitness goals. It's not an either-or scenario. Fasting and muscle preservation, like two dancers, can move in harmony, each enhancing the other's performance, leading to a display of strength, endurance, and grace.

Optimizing Workout Schedules Around Fasting

Mastering the art of integrating fasting with fitness requires a harmonious blend of knowledge, personal introspection, and a touch of experimentation. The concept isn't just to know when to exercise, but also to comprehend the physiology behind it. With this knowledge, one can tailor workouts to achieve desired results while enjoying the profound benefits of fasting.

The Body's Energy Systems in Perspective

Before diving into the best times to work out during a fast, it's crucial to understand the body's energy systems. The body derives energy from three primary systems:

Phosphagen System: This system provides immediate energy and is used for short, explosive activities, lasting about 10 seconds.

Glycolytic System: This system uses glucose, either from the blood or broken down from glycogen stored in muscles, to produce energy. Activities lasting from 10 seconds to 2 minutes, like a 400-meter sprint, predominantly use this system.

Oxidative System: This is the aerobic system, which relies on oxygen to convert glucose into energy. It's primarily used for sustained activities lasting longer than 2 minutes.

Energy Use and Fasting

In the absence of external food sources during a fast, the body strategically uses its energy stores. Glycogen from the liver and muscles is the first port of call, followed by fats when glycogen is depleted.

Fast-paced, High-intensity Workouts

High-intensity interval training (HIIT), sprints, and other fast-paced exercises rely heavily on the glycolytic system. Early into a fast, when glycogen stores remain intact, the body can effectively handle such workouts. However, as the fast progresses and glycogen diminishes, performance in high-intensity activities might decline.

For those practicing intermittent fasting, it could be beneficial to schedule these workouts during the early fasting hours or shortly before breaking the fast.

Endurance and Aerobic Workouts

Long, steady-state cardio exercises, such as jogging or cycling, predominantly use the oxidative system. Once the body depletes glycogen stores and enters a state of ketosis during fasting, it burns fat for energy. This state can be particularly advantageous for endurance athletes or those engaging in longer workout sessions. For those on extended fasts, these workouts might be best during the latter part of the fast when the body is in a fat-burning mode.

Strength and Resistance Training

Resistance training, such as weight lifting, primarily taps into the phosphagen and glycolytic systems. While it's possible to engage in strength training during a fasted state, it's essential to pay attention to the body's signals. If strength levels seem compromised, consider scheduling these sessions shortly before breaking the fast or after having a meal.

Recovery and Adaptation

While the focus is often on the workout itself, recovery is equally pivotal. During fasting, especially extended periods, recovery might take longer. Ensure adequate rest between sessions and consider incorporating practices like stretching, foam rolling, or even yoga to aid in muscle recovery.

The Influence of Circadian Rhythms

Beyond the type of exercise and the fasting state, the body's internal clock, or circadian rhythm, also plays a role. For many, physical performance peaks in the late afternoon to early evening, while early morning might see reduced performance. Aligning workout schedules with these natural rhythms, combined with the fasting state, can offer an optimized exercise experience.

Personal Variations: Listening to the Body

As much as science offers guidance, each individual's experience will differ. Some might find they can engage in high-intensity workouts even late into a fast, while others might struggle. The key lies in listening to one's body, noting how it responds, and tweaking schedules accordingly.

Hydration and Electrolyte Balance

During fasting, especially when combined with exercise, maintaining hydration is crucial. Electrolytes like sodium, potassium, and magnesium play vital roles in muscle function and energy production. Consider sipping on electrolyte-infused water, especially before intense workout sessions during a fast.

Final Musings

Merging fasting with fitness isn't a rigid science but an evolving journey. It's a dance where sometimes fasting leads and at other times, fitness takes the forefront. By understanding the body's energy systems, the nuances of different workouts, and the intricacies of fasting, one can choreograph a routine that's both effective and enjoyable. As with any journey, there will be moments of euphoria and times of challenge, but with each step, with each rep, with every fasting hour, one moves closer to a symphony of optimal health and unparalleled fitness.

Fasting and Endurance: A Match Made for Some

Endurance sports, by definition, challenge the boundaries of human potential. They're not just about strength or speed but the ability to sustain effort over prolonged periods. Marathons, triathlons, long-distance cycling, and ultra-running are all testaments to the spirit of endurance. However, introducing fasting into this equation brings a new dimension, sparking both curiosity and debate among athletes and enthusiasts.

Understanding Endurance at its Core

Endurance activities primarily tap into the oxidative system. Over time, as glycogen stores wane, the body has to shift towards other energy sources, primarily fats. This ability to switch between energy sources is pivotal for endurance athletes, ensuring they don't "hit the wall" during their activities.

Ketosis and Fat Adaptation: The Basics

When fasting or consuming a very low-carbohydrate diet, the body enters a state of ketosis. This state sees the liver breaking down fats into ketones, which can serve as an alternative fuel source, especially for the brain. This physiological adaptation, often termed "fat adaptation," can be of particular interest to endurance athletes. In essence, a fat-adapted athlete can tap into vast fat reserves for energy, potentially bypassing the dreaded wall many hit when glycogen stores run out.

The Pros of Combining Fasting with Endurance

Enhanced Fat Oxidation: Training in a fasted state can amplify the body's ability to utilize fat as fuel. Over time, this can improve endurance performance, especially in longer events where fat becomes the primary energy source.

Improved Metabolic Flexibility: Fasted training can enhance the body's ability to switch between fuel sources seamlessly, moving from glycogen to fat reserves without significant drops in performance.

Weight Management: For many endurance athletes, especially those in weight-sensitive sports, maintaining an optimal weight can enhance performance. Fasting, combined with regular training, can be an effective tool for weight management.

Mental Fortitude: Both fasting and endurance sports challenge the mind. Combining the two can cultivate a mental toughness that's invaluable, not just in sports but in life's many marathons.

The Potential Challenges

Initial Performance Drop: Especially for those new to fasting, there can be a temporary decline in performance. It takes time for the body to adjust and optimize its energy systems.

Recovery Considerations: Fasting can impact recovery times. Endurance athletes need to be especially attuned to their recovery needs, ensuring they provide the body with the necessary nutrients post-exercise.

Risk of Nutritional Deficiencies: Extended fasting or frequent fasted training sessions can lead to deficiencies in vital nutrients. It's essential to have a well-structured eating plan during feeding windows.

Listening to the Body: While many might experience benefits, fasting combined with intense endurance training isn't for everyone. Some might find it doesn't suit their physiology or goals.

Practical Tips for Integrating Fasting and Endurance

Start Slowly: If new to fasting, begin with shorter intermittent fasts, gradually increasing the duration over weeks or months.

Hydration is Key: With the loss of glycogen, the body also loses water. Ensure adequate hydration before, during, and after workouts.

Consider Electrolytes: Extended endurance activities, especially in hot conditions, can lead to significant electrolyte loss. Sipping on an electrolyte solution can help maintain balance.

Prioritize Recovery: Post-workout, especially after longer sessions, focus on consuming a balanced meal. This meal should have a mix of proteins, fats, and carbohydrates to aid recovery.

Test and Tweak: Before major events, test fasted training sessions to see how the body responds. This isn't the time for strict adherence to dogma but for listening to one's body and adjusting accordingly.

Seek Expert Guidance: Consider working with a nutritionist or coach familiar with both endurance sports and fasting. Their insights can be invaluable.

Real-life Insights: Stories from the Track

Julia, an ultra-marathon runner, began integrating fasting into her training regimen about a year ago. Initially drawn to fasting for its potential weight loss benefits, she soon discovered it offered her something more. "During my long runs, I found a new level of mental clarity. It wasn't just about the physical anymore. Fasting taught me the power of the mind," she shared.

Mark, a triathlete, had a slightly different experience. "I tried fasted training for a few months, but it didn't work for me. My performance dropped, and I felt fatigued. However, I still use intermittent fasting on my rest days. It's all about finding what works for you," he noted.

Embracing the Journey

Endurance is as much about the journey as it is about the destination. Introducing fasting into this journey is a deeply personal choice, one that can offer profound insights into one's body and mind. It's not about following trends but about discovering what truly resonates, what genuinely enhances the experience. For some, fasting and endurance might seem an unlikely pair, but for others, it might just be the match made in athletic heaven. As with all things in life, it's about exploration, understanding, and embracing the unique path that unfolds.

Strength Training and Fasting: Finding Synergy

Strength training, with its emphasis on building muscle mass, enhancing power, and increasing bone density, seems, at first glance, to be at odds with fasting. One focuses on fueling and rebuilding, while the other seemingly deprives the body of nutrients. However, when approached with knowledge and purpose, strength training and fasting can harmonize, offering a range of benefits that might be elusive when either is pursued in isolation.

Understanding the Dynamics of Muscle Growth

Muscle growth, or hypertrophy, occurs when muscle fibers experience damage during workouts and subsequently repair. This repair process requires adequate protein synthesis, which is influenced by both exercise and nutrient availability. The immediate thought is that fasting could hinder this process, given the lack of nutrients. However, the relationship between fasting, muscle growth, and strength training is more nuanced than it appears.

Benefits of Merging Strength Training with Fasting

Enhanced Human Growth Hormone (HGH) Production: Fasting can trigger an increase in the secretion of HGH, a critical hormone for muscle growth and overall health. This natural boost can be particularly beneficial for those engaged in strength training.

Improved Insulin Sensitivity: Strength training naturally improves insulin sensitivity. When combined with fasting, this effect is magnified, allowing muscles to uptake nutrients more effectively during the feeding window.

Increased Fat Oxidation: Training in a fasted state pushes the body to utilize stored fat for energy. This can be particularly advantageous for those looking to increase muscle definition.

Cellular Autophagy: Fasting activates autophagy, a cellular "clean-up" process. This can aid in the removal of damaged cells and proteins, promoting muscle health.

Potential Hurdles and Solutions

Energy Dips: Especially during the early stages, training in a fasted state can lead to reduced energy levels. It's crucial to gauge how the body reacts and adjust the intensity of workouts accordingly.

Muscle Catabolism Concerns: One of the primary concerns is that fasting might lead to muscle breakdown. However, short-term fasts, especially when paired with adequate protein intake during eating windows, are unlikely to result in significant muscle loss. BCAAs (Branched-Chain Amino Acids) can be consumed before a workout to prevent muscle breakdown.

Nutrient Timing: Post-workout nutrition becomes even more critical when strength training during a fast. Consuming protein-rich meals or shakes post-workout can optimize muscle repair and growth.

Strategies to Harmonize Strength Training and Fasting

Lean into Leucine: Leucine is an amino acid that plays a pivotal role in stimulating protein synthesis. Including leucine-rich foods like chicken, fish, beef, and soy during the eating window can support muscle growth.

Hydration Matters: Fasting can lead to dehydration, which in turn can affect muscle function. Stay adequately hydrated, especially on workout days.

Listen to the Body: Not every day will be optimal for intense strength training. It's essential to listen to the body's cues and adjust workout intensity accordingly.

Diversify Training: While strength training is the focus, incorporating flexibility and cardio workouts can enhance overall fitness and mitigate potential stress from fasted strength training sessions.

Seek Expertise: Just as one might consult a personal trainer for strength training tips, considering expert input on merging fasting with strength training can be invaluable.

Experiences from the Gym Floor

Elena, a fitness trainer, shares her journey: "When I first began combining fasting with my strength training regime, I was skeptical. But over time, I noticed not just changes in my physique but in my energy levels and recovery times. It's not always easy, but the benefits have been undeniable."

On the other hand, Tom, a bodybuilder, has a different tale: "I tried fasted workouts, but they weren't for me. I felt like I couldn't push as hard. However, I still integrate intermittent fasting on my rest days."

A Fusion of Strength and Restraint

At the intersection of strength training and fasting lies a delicate balance, a dance between exertion and restraint, building and healing. For those who find this synergy, the rewards extend beyond the visible. It's a testament to the body's resilience and adaptability, a journey of pushing boundaries while honoring limits. As always, the key lies not in blind adherence but in personalized exploration, adjusting, and adapting based on individual responses and goals. The strength lies not just in muscles but in the wisdom to find harmony in seemingly contrasting pursuits.

Rest, Recovery, and Fasting: The Trifecta of Wellness

Delving into the depths of human physiology reveals an intricate tapestry of processes, each harmoniously playing its part in sustaining life. Within this vast arena, three elements emerge as pillars of holistic wellness: rest, recovery, and fasting. While each has its individual merits, their combined effect on well-being can be transformative.

The Healing Power of Rest

Rest is not just the absence of activity; it's a potent, active state where the body undergoes repair, regeneration, and rejuvenation. The essence of rest isn't confined to sleep alone. It embodies moments of stillness, reflection, and detachment from the external hustle.

Sleep and Cellular Repair: During deep sleep phases, cells regenerate, toxins are flushed out, and vital hormones are produced. This makes sleep indispensable for overall health.

Mental Rest and Clarity: Disconnecting from constant stimuli, be it from electronic devices or demanding tasks, allows the mind to reset, fostering creativity, focus, and mental stamina.

Recovery: Beyond Muscle Repair

tossed around in fitness circles, often limited to muscle repair after intense workouts. While this is a critical component, recovery encapsulates more.

Muscle Recovery: After workouts, muscles experience microscopic tears. The healing of these tears results in muscle growth. Essential nutrients, especially protein, play a crucial role in this repair process.

Systemic Recovery: It's not just muscles that need recovery. Organs, especially the liver, the body's detox workhorse, require downtime from constant digestion and toxin processing.

Emotional and Psychological Recovery: Mental health is intertwined with physical well-being. Periods of relaxation, meditation, and disconnection can significantly boost emotional resilience.

Fasting: Nature's Reset Button

The practice of voluntarily refraining from food has roots in ancient traditions, often for spiritual reasons. Modern research, however, has unveiled a plethora of health benefits associated with strategic fasting.

Inducing Autophagy: This is the body's way of cleaning out damaged cells to regenerate newer, healthier ones. Fasting can amplify this process, promoting cellular health.

Enhancing Brain Function: Fasting triggers the release of BDNF (Brain-Derived Neurotrophic Factor), which supports cognitive function and reduces the risk of neurodegenerative diseases.

Balancing Insulin Levels: Regular fasting can stabilize insulin levels, reducing the risk of type 2 diabetes and other metabolic disorders.

Synergy of the Trio: A Closer Look

When rest, recovery, and fasting are approached as intertwined components, their collective impact on health is amplified.

Improved Immune Function: Adequate sleep, combined with the cellular cleanup from fasting, can enhance immune response, making the body more resilient to infections.

Optimal Hormone Production: Sleep is crucial for the secretion of hormones like melatonin and growth hormone. Fasting, in turn, optimizes insulin and ghrelin levels. Together, they ensure hormonal balance.

Enhanced Mood and Energy Levels: Quality rest and strategic fasting can boost energy levels and elevate mood by optimizing neurotransmitter levels.

Customizing the Trifecta for Individual Needs

While the benefits of combining rest, recovery, and fasting are evident, it's essential to tailor the approach based on individual requirements.

Listen to the Body: It provides constant feedback. Fatigue, mood swings, or prolonged muscle soreness are indicators that adjustments are needed.

Avoid Overtraining: Balancing intense workouts with adequate recovery and leveraging the benefits of fasting requires keen attention to prevent overtraining.

Flexible Fasting Protocols: While some might thrive on extended fasts, others might find intermittent fasting more suitable. The key is consistent experimentation and adaptation.

Narratives from Real Lives

Samantha, a yoga instructor, shares, "I've always emphasized rest and recovery in my regimen. But when I integrated fasting, the clarity, energy, and vitality I experienced were unparalleled."

Conversely, David, a marathon runner, observes, "While I found value in rest and recovery, fasting was a challenge. But with gradual incorporation, I've discovered a balance that enhances my performance."

Navigating the Path to Holistic Well-being

The voyage to optimal health is neither linear nor one-size-fits-all. It's a blend of understanding scientific principles and tuning into one's own body rhythms. Rest, recovery, and fasting, when approached with awareness and intent, can indeed be the guiding lights on this journey. As individuals across the globe embark on quests for better health, this trifecta stands as a testament to nature's wisdom, offering a roadmap to vitality, longevity, and holistic wellness. The journey might be personal, but the principles remain universal. Embrace them, and witness the metamorphosis into the best version of oneself.

8

Delicious Fasting: Nourishing Food Choices

Breaking the fast: Nutrient-dense choices

Embarking on a fasting journey is much like setting sail on calm seas. While the voyage demands patience, the true challenge often lies in anchoring back to shore, a parallel to breaking one's fast. The foods consumed upon completing a fast set the stage for the body's metabolic response, digestive rejuvenation, and overall well-being.

Understanding the Post-Fast Body

Upon concluding a fast, the body is in a heightened state of sensitivity. Digestive enzymes have taken a brief hiatus, the stomach lining is pristine, and the metabolic machinery is eager for fuel. Hence, the first foods introduced should be both gentle on the system and nutrient-rich.

Key Principles for Nutrient-Dense Choices

Gentleness is Paramount: The digestive system, after a period of rest, benefits from a gentle re-introduction to food. Heavy, greasy, or excessively spicy foods can overwhelm the system.

Prioritize Hydration: Often, the body's need for hydration supersedes its hunger. Initiating the break with hydrating foods ensures optimal cellular function and prepares the digestive tract for solid foods.

Embrace Whole Foods: Nature, in its infinite wisdom, offers foods that are complete packages of macro and micronutrients. Whole foods, devoid of artificial additives, are the ideal candidates to grace the post-fast plate.

Foods That Shine Post-Fast

1. **Bone Broth:** This elixir, simmered for hours, is rich in collagen, amino acids, and minerals. Its gelatin content soothes the digestive tract, making it an excellent choice to break longer fasts.
2. **Steamed Vegetables:** Lightly steamed non-starchy vegetables, like spinach, zucchini, or asparagus, are easy on the stomach. They provide essential vitamins, minerals, and fiber, aiding in gentle bowel movement.
3. **Fresh Fruits:** Water-rich fruits like melon, berries, or peaches can hydrate and offer fructose, a simple sugar, for a quick energy boost. However, it's essential to gauge individual tolerance, especially for those sensitive to sugar spikes.
4. **Nuts and Seeds:** Soaked almonds, chia seeds, or flaxseeds can be introduced as the body gets accustomed to food post-fast. They're dense in essential fats, proteins, and minerals.
5. **Fermented Foods:** Yogurt, kefir, or fermented vegetables introduce beneficial bacteria to the gut, fortifying the microbiome and aiding digestion.

Crafting the Perfect Post-Fast Plate

When imagining a post-fast meal, envision a plate abundant in colors, textures, and nutrients. Here's a sample plate that embodies nutrient-density:

A Warm Cup of Bone Broth: A sip of this warms the system, prepping it for the feast ahead.

A Rainbow Salad: Spinach, cherry tomatoes, red bell peppers, sprinkled with soaked chia seeds, dressed with olive oil, and a dash of lemon.

A Side of Protein: A soft-boiled egg or a portion of grilled tofu, providing essential amino acids.

A Dollop of Fermented Goodness: A spoonful of yogurt or a few fermented carrot sticks.

While this plate serves as inspiration, individual preferences, dietary restrictions, and the length of the fast can dictate variations. The essence, however, remains consistent: prioritize nutrient density.

Listening to Body Signals

While guidelines provide direction, the body's cues are paramount. Some might feel satiated with just a cup of broth, while others might need a more substantial plate. Some might resonate with fruits, while others might gravitate towards vegetables. The key lies in mindfulness, patience, and attuning to one's unique rhythms.

Stories from the Fasting Community

Lila, an intermittent fasting enthusiast, shares, "Breaking my fast has become a sacred ritual. I often start with a warm cup of herbal tea, followed by a fruit. The sense of gratitude I feel with that first bite is unparalleled."

On the other hand, Raj, who practices extended fasting, observes, "Bone broth has been my go-to. It not only satiates but also feels healing. As I progress, I introduce soft foods, always ensuring I'm in tune with my body's signals."

The Dance of Nutrients and Taste

While nutrient density is the cornerstone of breaking a fast, the joy derived from savoring flavors amplifies the experience. It's this delicate dance between nutrients and taste that transforms the act of eating post-fast from a mere task to a delightful celebration.

As fasting voyages become integral to many health journeys, understanding the art and science of breaking them becomes crucial. The foods chosen in this pivotal phase can either augment the benefits of the fast or diminish them. With mindfulness, knowledge, and a dash of culinary creativity, one can craft post-fast meals that not only nourish but also delight. And as the journey of 'Her Fast, Her Freedom' unfolds, this delicate balance between sustenance and pleasure stands as a beacon, illuminating paths to holistic well-being.

Hydrating adequately: Beyond plain water

Hydration is often reduced to the mere act of drinking water. It's much more nuanced, especially when it comes to the fasting lifestyle tailored for women. As our body transitions through different phases of the menstrual cycle, its hydration needs, too, undergo subtle changes. Staying adequately hydrated during a fast is not just about quenching thirst; it's about nourishing the body, supporting detoxification, and ensuring smooth cellular processes.

Water, while irreplaceably vital, doesn't solely fulfill our hydration requirements. The female body, with its intricate hormonal dance and metabolic uniqueness, demands more than just plain water, especially during fasting.

Electrolyte balance during fasting

When fasting, insulin levels decrease, which prompts the kidneys to excrete more sodium. While this can be beneficial in terms of reducing bloating and managing blood pressure, it can also lead to an electrolyte imbalance. Incorporating beverages rich in electrolytes can help maintain this balance. Think coconut water, a natural electrolyte booster, or broths that can supply sodium and other minerals.

Herbal infusions: More than flavor

Beyond the calming effects of chamomile or the stimulating zest of peppermint, herbal teas play a significant role in hydration during fasting. Dandelion tea, for example, acts as a gentle diuretic, aiding in detoxification. Red raspberry leaf tea, considered a women's herb, can be particularly beneficial for uterine health. Nettle tea, abundant in minerals, aids in replenishing lost nutrients during fasting.

Fruits and their hydrating power

While consuming fruits during a fast isn't always recommended, particularly in strict water fasts, one can't overlook their hydrating potential for the times you're not fasting. Fruits like watermelon, cucumber, and strawberries have high water content. They not only hydrate but also provide essential vitamins and minerals, supporting overall well-being.

Hydratioand skin health

For many women, fasting has an aesthetic angle as well - radiant skin. While the act of fasting promotes cellular autophagy, leading to rejuvenated skin cells, hydration plays an equally pivotal role. When adequately hydrated, the skin appears plumper, wrinkles are less noticeable, and there's a natural glow that no makeup can replicate. Infused waters, with slices of fruits or herbs, can add a dimension of skin-loving nutrients to your hydration routine.

Hydrating for hormonal health

The hormonal symphony in a woman's body requires adequate hydration for optimal functioning. Water helps in the smooth transportation of hormones to their destination in the body. During the luteal phase, where some women experience bloating and breast tenderness, proper hydration can mitigate these symptoms.

Fasting and thirst perception

One peculiar aspect of fasting, particularly prolonged ones, is the altered thirst perception. Some women report not feeling as thirsty as they usually do. This can lead to unintentional dehydration. It's paramount to stay cognizant of hydration needs, even if the body isn't screaming for water. Setting reminders or having a water schedule can be beneficial in such scenarios.

Bone broths and their dual role

Bone broths are not just flavorsome but are nutritional powerhouses. Rich in collagen, they support joint health, an often-overlooked aspect of women's health. They also provide a plethora of minerals, ensuring that the body doesn't feel depleted during a fast. Moreover, the warm and soothing nature of broths can be particularly comforting during a fast, making the journey more palatable.

Mindful hydration

Just as we emphasize mindfulness in eating, hydration, too, deserves such focused attention. Paying heed to the body's signals, understanding its unique needs during various phases of the menstrual cycle, and adjusting hydration strategies accordingly can make a world of difference. It's not just about drinking more but drinking right.

Every droplet of water, every sip of tea, and every mouthful of broth is a step towards a more nourished, balanced, and vibrant self. As women, as we navigate the world of fasting, understanding the profound role of hydration becomes indispensable. It's not just about quenching thirst; it's about quenching the body's innate desire for balance, wellness, and vitality.

Keto and fasting: A dynamic duo for fat loss?

The ketogenic diet, often referred to as keto, is a low-carbohydrate, high-fat dietary approach. With carbohydrates limited, the body shifts its energy source from glucose to ketones, leading to a metabolic state called ketosis. Fasting, on the other hand, is the voluntary abstention from consuming food for specific periods. At a first glance, the synergistic relationship between keto and fasting appears evident, both aiming to tap into the body's fat reserves for energy. But is this combination the golden ticket for women seeking fat loss?

Understanding the Ketogenic Diet

At the core of the ketogenic diet is the idea of transforming the body into a fat-burning machine. By drastically reducing carbohydrate intake, the body runs out of its preferred energy source, glucose. In response, the liver begins breaking down fatty acids into ketones, which then serve as an alternative fuel.

Keto's Relationship with Female Metabolism

While men and women can both benefit from keto, the female metabolism has unique nuances. Hormonal fluctuations throughout the menstrual cycle can affect how women respond to a carbohydrate-restricted diet. For some, the luteal phase, marked by a spike in progesterone, might demand a slightly higher carb intake to stave off mood swings or cravings.

Entering Ketosis: The Transition Phase

Transitioning to a ketogenic diet isn't always smooth. The initial days can be marked by symptoms collectively termed the "keto flu." This includes fatigue, headache, dizziness, and irritability. As the body adjusts to burning fat for fuel, these symptoms typically subside.

Fasting: A Natural Ketosis Booster

The act of fasting naturally propels the body towards ketosis. As the body exhausts its glucose reserves, it turns to ketones for energy. Therefore, someone practicing intermittent fasting or engaging in extended fasts may find themselves in a mild state of ketosis, even if they aren't following a strict ketogenic diet.

Keto and Fasting: Amplifying Fat Loss

When combined, keto and fasting can accelerate the body's transition into ketosis. Being already adapted to using ketones for energy on a ketogenic diet can make fasting experiences more manageable. Likewise, regular fasting can make maintaining ketosis on non-fasting days more effortless.

Protein: The Unsung Hero

Amidst the focus on fats and carbs, protein deserves equal attention. Essential for muscle repair, growth, and maintenance, protein becomes especially crucial for women engaging in both keto and fasting. This ensures muscle preservation even as the body taps into fat reserves.

Potential Challenges and Considerations

Keto and fasting, while potentially powerful, are not without challenges. Ensuring micronutrient adequacy becomes crucial as carb-rich fruits, vegetables, and grains are limited. Electrolyte imbalances might arise, necessitating supplementation or dietary adjustments.

Women with thyroid issues or adrenal fatigue should approach this combination with caution. A drastic reduction in carbohydrate intake can sometimes exacerbate these conditions. It's imperative to monitor symptoms and work closely with a healthcare professional.

Customizing the Approach

There's no one-size-fits-all. Some women might thrive on a strict ketogenic diet combined with regular fasting, while others might need occasional carb-ups. Listening to one's body, being open to adjustments, and prioritizing well-being over strict adherence to any dietary doctrine is key.

Keto-Friendly Fast-Breaking Foods

Breaking a fast with keto-friendly foods can be both nourishing and delightful. Avocado, with its rich potassium content, is an excellent choice. Bone broths, offering both protein and minerals, can be both soothing and nutritious. Nuts and seeds, like almonds or chia seeds, can provide a satiating combination of fats, protein, and fiber.

Are Keto and Fasting the Ultimate Duo for Every Woman?

While the benefits of combining keto and fasting are evident, it's essential to acknowledge individuality. What works wonders for one might not be optimal for another. The goal isn't just fat loss but holistic health, vitality, and a sense of well-being. Any dietary approach, no matter how popular or effective, should be a means to that end.

Plant-based fasting: A viable option

The plant-based movement, anchored in the myriad health, environmental, and ethical benefits of consuming plants over animal products, has gained significant momentum. Simultaneously, fasting continues its upward trajectory in popularity. Merging the two may seem like an uncharted territory, but the landscape of plant-based fasting presents a promising, nutrient-rich, and compassionate approach to health and well-being.

Defining Plant-Based

At its core, a plant-based diet revolves around whole foods derived from plants, including vegetables, fruits, grains, nuts, seeds, and legumes, while minimizing or eliminating animal products.

Plant-Based Diet: A Spectrum

Plant-based diets encompass various degrees, from vegetarians, who may consume dairy or eggs, to vegans, who strictly avoid all animal-derived products. There's also a focus on whole foods, which differentiates a health-centric plant-based diet from a diet simply devoid of animal products but potentially full of processed foods.

Nutrient Density: The Plant-Based Advantage

One of the hallmarks of a plant-based diet is its nutrient density. Leafy greens, berries, nuts, and seeds are packed with vitamins, minerals, antioxidants, and phytonutrients. This nutrient density can be particularly advantageous during fasting periods. When the eating window is limited, maximizing nutrient intake becomes paramount.

Protein and Plant-Based Fasting

One of the common concerns around plant-based diets revolves around protein. However, with a little planning, meeting protein needs is feasible. Legumes, tofu, tempeh, edamame, quinoa, and hemp seeds are potent protein sources. When breaking a fast, these protein sources can aid in muscle repair and growth.

Fats in the Plant Kingdom

Healthy fats are crucial, more so in the context of fasting, for satiety and hormonal balance. Avocados, olives, nuts, seeds, and coconuts are rich in monounsaturated and polyunsaturated fats. Flaxseeds and walnuts provide a plant-based source of Omega-3 fatty acids, vital for brain health and inflammation control.

Carbohydrates: Fueling Fasts the Plant-Based Way

Whole food sources of carbohydrates, like sweet potatoes, quinoa, fruits, and legumes, provide sustained energy. These complex carbs are rich in fiber, ensuring digestive health, and steady blood sugar levels, particularly essential when transitioning out of a fast.

Plant-Based Hydration Options

Hydration during fasting isn't merely about water. Herbal teas, vegetable broths, or simple infusions with cucumber, mint, or berries can offer both hydration and a dose of nutrients. Coconut water, in moderation, can be a natural electrolyte replenisher.

Micronutrient Considerations

Certain nutrients, typically found in animal products, need extra attention in a plant-based regime. Vitamin B12, Vitamin D, Iron, Calcium, Omega-3, and Iodine may require conscious planning, fortified foods, or supplementation.

Gut Health and Plant-Based Fasting

A plant-based diet, with its emphasis on fiber, can be immensely beneficial for gut health. Fermented foods, like sauerkraut, kimchi, and plant-based yogurts, introduce beneficial bacteria to the gut, fortifying the microbiome, especially essential after a fasting period.

Satiety and Plant-Based Foods

Contrary to misconceptions, plant-based foods can be incredibly satiating. Foods like chia seeds, avocados, or legumes are not only nutrient-rich but also ensure feelings of fullness, which can be particularly helpful when practicing intermittent fasting.

Plant-Based Fasting: Ethical and Environmental Dimensions

Beyond personal health, plant-based fasting also treads on the path of compassion. It reduces the demand for animal farming, known for its environmental and ethical concerns. Lower carbon footprint, reduced water usage, and a step away from factory farming practices align the individual's health journey with broader planetary wellness.

Creating a Plant-Based Fast-Breaking Menu

Fast-breaking foods should be gentle on the digestive system while providing ample nutrients. A smoothie with spinach, berries, flaxseeds, and almond milk; a salad with mixed greens, roasted chickpeas, avocado, and a tahini dressing; or a simple lentil soup can be both nourishing and satisfying.

Incorporating Diversity: The Key to Nutrient Sufficiency

A varied diet ensures a spectrum of nutrients. Rotating between different grains, legumes, vegetables, and fruits is not just a treat for the palate but a strategy to ensure comprehensive nutrition.

Plant-based fasting, while requiring some planning, emerges as a viable, compassionate, and nutrient-rich approach. It aligns individual well-being with broader ecological and ethical considerations. As more women explore fasting's transformative power, plant-based fasting presents a path that's both nourishing for the body and kind to the planet.

Recipe inspirations for fast-breaking meals

The act of breaking a fast is a significant one, symbolizing not just the end of a period of abstaining but also the beginning of nourishing the body. The meals chosen to break a fast can set the tone for the rest of the day, both in terms of nutrition and overall well-being. Here, we delve deep into an assortment of inspired recipes tailored for fast-breaking that ensures a gentle, nourishing reintroduction of food.

Gentle Green Smoothie

Ingredients:
Handful of spinach
1 small cucumber, sliced
Half an avocado
1 tablespoon chia seeds
1 cup almond milk or any plant-based milk
1/2 lemon, juiced

Method:

Blend all ingredients until smooth. This smoothie offers hydration, essential fats, and protein, making it an ideal choice for breaking a fast.

Warm Quinoa and Roasted Veggie Salad

Ingredients:

1 cup cooked quinoa

Assorted vegetables (zucchini, bell peppers, cherry tomatoes)

1 tablespoon olive oil

Salt, to taste

A handful of fresh parsley, chopped

1 tablespoon lemon juice

Method:

Roast the veggies in olive oil until tender. Mix with quinoa, parsley, and lemon juice. This dish offers a dose of complex carbohydrates and essential micronutrients.

Creamy Coconut and Lentil Soup

Ingredients:

1 cup lentils, washed and soaked

400ml can of coconut milk

1 onion, finely chopped

2 cloves of garlic, minced

1 tablespoon olive oil

Salt and pepper, to taste

Method:

In a pot, sauté onions and garlic in olive oil until translucent. Add lentils and enough water to cover them. Simmer until lentils are tender. Add coconut milk, salt, and pepper. Serve warm.

Berry Bliss Chia Pudding

Ingredients:

   3 tablespoons chia seeds

   1 cup almond milk or any plant-based milk

   A mix of berries (blueberries, raspberries, strawberries)

   1 tablespoon maple syrup or sweetener of choice

Method:

Mix chia seeds with almond milk and let it sit for a couple of hours or overnight until it forms a gel-like consistency. Layer with berries and sweeten with maple syrup.

Almond Butter and Banana Wrap

Ingredients:

   Whole grain wrap or tortilla

   2 tablespoons almond butter

   1 banana, sliced

Method:

Spread almond butter on the wrap. Place banana slices and roll. This provides an instant energy boost with good fats, protein, and carbs.

Stuffed Avocados

Ingredients:

   2 ripe avocados, halved and pitted

   1 cup chickpeas, boiled and mashed

Lemon juice
Salt and pepper, to taste
Cherry tomatoes, sliced
Olive oil
Method:
Mix mashed chickpeas with lemon juice, salt, pepper, and cherry tomatoes. Fill avocado halves with this mixture. Drizzle with olive oil. A meal rich in healthy fats and protein.

Golden Turmeric Tofu Scramble

Ingredients:
  200g firm tofu, crumbled
  1 tablespoon turmeric powder
  1 small onion, chopped
  A handful of spinach
  Salt, to taste
  1 tablespoon olive oil
Method:
Sauté onions in olive oil. Add crumbled tofu, turmeric, and salt. Once cooked, add spinach and cook till wilted. A protein-rich dish with the benefits of turmeric.

Refreshing Cucumber Mint Salad

Ingredients:
  2 cucumbers, sliced
  Handful of mint leaves, chopped
  Lemon juice
  Salt and pepper, to taste
Method:

Mix all ingredients. This hydrating salad is perfect for replenishing fluids post-fast.

Chocolate Protein Energy Bites

Ingredients:
  1 cup dates, pitted
  2 tablespoons cocoa powder
  1/2 cup oats
  1/2 cup almonds
Method:
Blend all ingredients in a food processor until it forms a dough-like consistency. Shape into balls. A quick energy booster.

Soothing Herbal Tea Infusion

Ingredients:
  1 teaspoon chamomile flowers
  1 teaspoon fennel seeds
  Hot water
Method:
Steep chamomile and fennel in hot water for 5 minutes. A calming drink to complement the fast-breaking meal.

These recipes are not just about the ingredients or the nutrition they provide; they symbolize a deeper connection to one's body, understanding its needs, and nurturing it with love and care. Crafting a meal to break a fast is a ritual, a way to say thank you to the body for its resilience and strength. As fasting journeys continue, these recipes serve as a guide, a starting point to explore, innovate, and personalize according to individual needs and tastes.

9

Mindful Fasting: The Psychological Journey

Fostering a positive mindset for fasting success

Embarking on a fasting journey is more than just refraining from food. It is a powerful undertaking that encompasses both physical and mental disciplines. In many ways, the mental discipline required is even more crucial than the physical. The mind plays a pivotal role, setting the stage for success or defeat. Here, we delve into the art and science of fostering a positive mindset, a tool instrumental in achieving fasting success.

Recognize the Power of Thought

Every achievement begins as a thought. Humans are unique in their capacity for self-reflection and foresight. By harnessing the power of positive thought, one can lay a foundation of strength and determination. Regularly visualizing successful fasting experiences can pave the way for actual success.

Meditation and Mindfulness

Meditation is not merely a practice; it's a journey inwards. It allows introspection and a profound connection with one's inner self. By practicing meditation, one can enhance awareness and better navigate the challenges posed during fasting. Mindfulness, on the other hand, is about being present, fully experiencing each moment. Instead of dreading the hours until the next meal, practicing mindfulness encourages one to relish the sensations and experiences of the fasting state.

Affirmations and Self-talk

Words hold power. The way one talks to oneself can uplift or defeat. Crafting positive affirmations specific to the fasting journey can act as an anchor during challenging moments. Some examples include "I am stronger than my cravings" or "Each moment of fasting brings me closer to my goals." Repeating these affirmations, especially during vulnerable times, can offer solace and strength.

Educate and Empower

Knowledge dispels fear. Understanding the physiological processes that occur during fasting can be empowering. By knowing the benefits, like autophagy and improved insulin sensitivity, one can view fasting not as deprivation but as a gift to the body. Engage with credible sources, attend seminars, or read books on fasting. The more one knows, the more confidence one gains.

Visual Aids

Creating a vision board can be a transformative tool. Pin up images, quotes, or any visual cues that inspire and align with fasting goals. Place this board in a visible area. It serves as a constant reminder of the purpose and the potential of the fasting journey.

Journaling the Journey

Writing has therapeutic properties. Maintaining a fasting journal can offer insights into patterns, triggers, and progress. Pen down thoughts, feelings, and experiences during fasting. Over time, this journal can serve as a testament to one's resilience and progress.

Surround with Support

Human beings are inherently social creatures. Engaging with a community or even just one supportive individual can make a significant difference. Share fasting goals with friends or family, or consider joining a fasting support group. Sharing experiences, challenges, and successes with others creates a sense of camaraderie and encouragement.

Celebrate Small Wins

Fasting is a marathon, not a sprint. Instead of just waiting for that one big goal, celebrate the small milestones along the way. Whether it's successfully completing a 16-hour fast or resisting a particular craving, each achievement is a step towards the larger goal.

Embrace Challenges as Lessons

No journey is devoid of challenges. Instead of perceiving them as setbacks, view them as lessons. Each challenge offers an opportunity to learn, grow, and fortify one's determination. By adopting this mindset, challenges transform from roadblocks into stepping stones.

Focus on Holistic Well-being

Fasting is just one piece of the wellness puzzle. Incorporate other facets of well-being, be it regular exercise, adequate sleep, or engaging in hobbies. When one feels good overall, maintaining a positive mindset towards fasting becomes more effortless.

Practice Gratitude

Gratitude has the power to shift perspectives. Instead of focusing on what's being abstained from, focus on the myriad benefits and the privilege of being able to choose fasting for health. A daily gratitude practice, listing things one is thankful for, can create a ripple effect of positivity.

Fostering a positive mindset is akin to nurturing a garden. With consistent effort, patience, and care, it flourishes. The mindset cultivated not only propels one towards fasting success but also permeates other areas of life. It becomes a beacon, guiding through challenges, illuminating possibilities, and fostering growth. As the fasting journey unfolds, let this positive mindset be the trusted companion, illuminating the path towards holistic well-being.

Overcoming Fears and Anxiety Associated with Fasting

Fasting has been interwoven into the fabric of human history, a practice spanning cultures, religions, and epochs. Yet, in the landscape of modern lifestyles and conveniences, fasting often emerges draped in apprehensions, uncertainties, and anxieties. Navigating these emotions is crucial, for they form the silent undertones that can either support or hinder a fasting journey.

Understanding the Roots of Fear

At its core, fear serves as a protective mechanism. Millennia of evolution have hardwired humans to seek nourishment and avoid starvation. In this context, fasting may trigger alarms in the brain, hinting at potential threats. Remember, it's not just about the physical body; the mind perceives risk, especially when presented with a shift as significant as abstaining from food.

Yet, much of modern fear around fasting is not purely primal. Societal influences, misinformation, and personal experiences weave a complex web. From comments like "You'll waste away!" to concerns about energy depletion or muscle loss, external voices amplify internal worries.

Differentiating between Fear and Caution

Caution and fear might seem synonymous, but they stand on opposite ends of the spectrum. Caution is an informed, conscious decision to approach situations with prudence. Fear, on the other hand, is a primal, often irrational, response. While caution is beneficial, guiding one to undertake fasting with knowledge and preparation, fear can be paralyzing.

Countering Myths with Knowledge

Arming oneself with accurate information is paramount. When confronted with a fear, ask: Is this fact or fiction? Many concerns surrounding fasting originate from misconceptions.

Starvation Mode Myth: One common myth is that fasting sends the body into 'starvation mode,' slowing metabolism and hoarding fat. In reality, short-term fasting can boost metabolic rate and promote fat burning.

Loss of Muscle Mass: Another fear is the rapid loss of muscle. The body prioritizes using fat for energy during a fast. While prolonged fasting without proper preparation may impact muscle, short-term and intermittent fasting have minimal effect.

Energy Depletion: Many anticipate a significant energy dip. In contrast, once the body transitions from using glucose to fat as its primary energy source, many report heightened clarity and vigor.

Embracing a Support System

An echoing concern or a lingering doubt shared might find resolution or at least lessening in intensity. Joining fasting communities, seeking the counsel of experienced fasters, or engaging with professionals can make the journey smoother. These platforms offer an avenue to voice apprehensions, seek solutions, and gain reassurance.

The Role of Gradual Introduction

Diving headlong into a prolonged fast can be overwhelming. Starting with shorter fasts, such as intermittent fasting, provides the body and mind time to adjust. These smaller commitments serve dual purposes. Physiologically, they prepare the body. Psychologically, they offer tangible experiences to counter fears.

Journaling the Journey

Documenting experiences, feelings, and progress is therapeutic. It not only offers a means to reflect but serves as a tangible record of one's journey. On days marred by doubt, flipping through past entries can provide perspective and encouragement.

Meditative Practices and Mindfulness

Meditation is not just an act but a state of being, a heightened consciousness where one is acutely aware yet detached. Incorporating meditation into fasting can help in managing anxieties. Simple breathing exercises can offer solace during moments of intense doubt. Mindfulness, the art of being present, can further aid in distinguishing between actual physical discomfort and mental apprehensions.

Affirmations and Visualization

The power of the mind is immense. Positive affirmations, repeated with conviction, can reshape thought patterns. Visualizing the end goals, whether they're health-related, spiritual, or both, can serve as powerful motivators. By visualizing success and the benefits of fasting, the journey becomes more about the destination and less about the hurdles.

Recognizing the Difference between Mental and Physical Signals

The body possesses its language. A growling stomach, a slight headache, or dizziness – these are signals. Yet, it's essential to differentiate between actual physical discomfort and mental projections. A passing thought about food can escalate into a perceived intense hunger pang if not checked. Training the mind to recognize and respond appropriately to these signals is essential.

Setting Clear Intentions

Why fast? The reasons are myriad, from detoxification, spiritual connection, weight loss, to metabolic health improvement. Clear intentions provide a roadmap. When fear sets in, revisiting these core reasons can serve as a compass, realigning focus.

Educating the Skeptics

Well-meaning family and friends, not familiar with the nuances of fasting, might project their fears. It's essential to differentiate between genuine concern and mere projection. Offering information and sharing the science and benefits behind fasting can sometimes assuage their worries, making them allies in the journey.

Accepting Fear as a Part of the Journey

Fear is human. It's natural. Instead of suppressing or battling it, recognizing and embracing it as a part of the journey can be liberating. With each fast, with each victory, however small, the looming shadows of doubt recede, replaced by confidence and a deeper understanding of one's body and psyche.

The journey of fasting, especially in its initial stages, is as much psychological as it is physical. By equipping oneself with knowledge, seeking support, and employing mindfulness techniques, the chasms of fear can be bridged. On the other side lies a realm of newfound freedom, health, and self-awareness - a realm where each woman finds not just her fast, but also her freedom.

Body image and fasting: A double-edged sword?

Body image is a highly personal and often sensitive subject for many, especially women. The standards set by society, the media, peers, and sometimes even family can significantly influence how one views and feels about their body. And in the realm of fasting, the topic of body image becomes even more poignant.

Fasting has been hailed as a method of weight and fat loss, making it attractive for many who aspire to align with societal beauty standards. This alignment with weight loss has inevitably tied fasting to the concept of body image. On one side, fasting offers the promise of a healthier, leaner physique, and a tool for achieving aesthetic goals. On the other side, it can inadvertently become a vehicle for perpetuating unhealthy body standards and exacerbating negative self-perception.

When women embark on a fasting journey with the primary goal of achieving a particular body aesthetic, they may sometimes place undue stress on themselves. They might equate their self-worth with their ability to adhere to a fasting regimen or with the number on the scale. This way of thinking can potentially lead to obsessive behaviors, disordered eating patterns, and even mental health issues.

However, the relationship between fasting and body image is not inherently negative. For many women, fasting serves as an avenue of self-discovery, empowerment, and a way to foster a healthier relationship with their bodies. Here's a deeper look into the complexities of this relationship:

1. Empowerment and Autonomy:

Fasting allows women to take control of their eating patterns and health. It provides a sense of autonomy, where one decides when to eat and when to fast. This control can be incredibly empowering, helping women to feel more connected with their bodies, listening to its signals, and nourishing it appropriately.

2. Breaking Free from Societal Pressure:

While some may begin fasting to align with societal beauty standards, the journey often evolves. Many women report that as they continue fasting, their focus shifts from external validation to internal well-being. The process of fasting can be a way to break free from societal pressures and cultivate a more genuine self-appreciation.

3. The Trap of Perfectionism:

However, it's essential to recognize that fasting can sometimes lead to perfectionistic tendencies. The desire to follow a fasting regimen perfectly can become overwhelming. If one breaks their fast earlier than planned or indulges a bit more during the eating window, it might lead to feelings of guilt or inadequacy. This pressure to be perfect can further distort body image and self-perception.

4. Physical Changes Beyond Aesthetics:

While fasting can lead to weight loss and changes in physique, its benefits are far beyond aesthetics. Improved energy levels, better mental clarity, hormonal balance, and enhanced overall well-being are some of the profound benefits that often accompany fasting. Recognizing and valuing these changes can help shift the focus from purely physical appearance to overall health and vitality.

5. The Importance of Community:

The fasting journey can be more manageable and fulfilling when undertaken within a supportive community. Engaging with others who are on similar paths can provide encouragement, diverse perspectives, and shared experiences. These interactions can reinforce the idea that body image is multifaceted and that everyone's journey is unique.

6. Intuitive Eating and Fasting:

One of the most transformative aspects of fasting can be the development of intuitive eating habits. As women fast, many learn to listen more closely to their body's hunger and satiety cues. This heightened awareness can help in fostering a healthier relationship with food and, by extension, a more positive body image.

7. Seeking Balance:

Like any tool, fasting should be used with care and mindfulness. It's essential to recognize when it may be causing more harm than good. If feelings of anxiety, negative self-worth, or obsessive behaviors start to emerge, it might be time to reassess the approach to fasting.

In the realm of body image, fasting is neither a hero nor a villain. Its impact largely depends on individual perspectives, motivations, and experiences. Fasting can be a journey of self-love, empowerment, and health, but it's essential to approach it with mindfulness, self-compassion, and a broader perspective that extends beyond physical appearance.

As we delve further into the psychological aspects of fasting, it becomes evident that the journey is as much about the mind as it is about the body. Embracing mindfulness practices, celebrating small victories, and consistently checking in with oneself can pave the way for a fulfilling and holistic fasting experience.

Mindfulness practices to enhance fasting experiences

Mindfulness, at its core, is the practice of being present, fully engaged with whatever we're doing, free from distraction or judgment, and with a soft and open mind. When interwoven with fasting, mindfulness can profoundly enhance the experience, turning it from a mere dietary routine into a holistic journey of self-discovery, balance, and well-being.

1. Understanding the Core of Mindfulness in Fasting:

At the outset, it's vital to grasp that mindfulness is not just a tool to make fasting easier, but a paradigm shift in how one approaches life, including one's relationship with food. It teaches acceptance, patience, and understanding, traits that are immensely beneficial when navigating the challenges of fasting.

2. Starting with Breath:

One of the most foundational practices in mindfulness is focusing on one's breath. During fasting, especially when hunger pangs hit, taking deep, controlled breaths can provide an immediate sense of calm. This conscious breathing serves as a reminder that hunger, like all sensations, is temporary and will pass.

3. Body Scan Meditation:

This is a practice where attention is slowly shifted to different parts of the body, observing sensations without judgment. During fasting, body scan meditation can help in tuning into the body's true needs versus its wants. It allows for the differentiation between true hunger and the mere desire to eat, often stemming from boredom or emotional triggers.

4. Mindful Eating:

When it's time to break the fast, it's easy to rush into consuming food. However, a mindful approach emphasizes savoring every bite, chewing slowly, and truly appreciating the nourishment food provides. This not only enhances digestion but also deepens gratitude for the meal, making the act of eating a more fulfilling experience.

5. Observing Hunger Without Action:

An integral part of mindfulness during fasting is observing sensations without reacting. This means acknowledging hunger, sitting with it, understanding its nuances, but not immediately seeking to satiate it. Over time, this practice can reduce the anxiety associated with hunger and cultivate a deeper understanding of the body's signals.

6. Journaling:

Documenting the fasting journey through a mindfulness lens can be transformative. Journaling allows for introspection, helping one to identify patterns, emotional triggers, and moments of growth. It serves as both a record and a tool for reflection, offering insights that can guide future fasting experiences.

7. Gratitude Practices:

While fasting, it's beneficial to cultivate gratitude, not just for food, but for the body's resilience, the clarity of mind, and the opportunity to grow spiritually and emotionally. A simple gratitude practice involves listing three things one is thankful for every day. Over time, this shifts focus from what is lacking or desired to what is already present and cherished.

8. Guided Meditations:

For those new to mindfulness, guided meditations can be an excellent starting point. Numerous apps and online platforms offer meditations specifically tailored for fasting or cultivating a healthy relationship with food. These guided sessions provide structure and guidance, helping individuals navigate the journey more seamlessly.

9. Embracing Silence:

In today's constantly connected world, silence has become a rarity. Yet, it is in these silent moments that one can truly connect with oneself. Designating periods of silence, devoid of gadgets or distractions, can amplify the benefits of fasting, giving the mind the much-needed respite it deserves.

10. Setting Intentions:

Each fasting period can begin with a set intention. It might be as simple as aiming for clarity, healing, or even understanding a particular emotion. Setting an intention turns the fasting period into a purpose-driven experience, providing motivation and a clear direction.

11. Progressive Relaxation:

This technique involves tensing and then slowly relaxing different muscle groups in the body. It can be particularly beneficial when fasting, as it not only aids relaxation but also diverts attention from hunger, channeling it towards the act of relaxation.

12. Mindful Movement:

Physical activity doesn't have to be rigorous exercise. Gentle, mindful movements like tai chi, qigong, or even simple stretching can be incorporated during fasting. These movements, when done with attention and intention, can enhance energy flow, alleviate physical discomfort associated with fasting, and offer a sense of grounding.

13. Cultivating Non-Judgment:

Not every fasting experience will be the same. There will be days when it feels more challenging, and others when it feels almost effortless. Mindfulness teaches non-judgment, meaning each experience is observed as it is, without labeling it as 'good' or 'bad'. This non-judgmental stance is crucial, especially on difficult fasting days, ensuring that one isolated experience doesn't derail the entire journey.

14. Affirmations:

Positive affirmations, when repeated consistently, can reshape beliefs and attitudes. During fasting, affirmations like "I am nourishing my body", "I am stronger than my cravings", or "Every moment of fasting brings me closer to balance" can serve as anchors, offering strength and perspective.

15. Group Mindfulness Sessions:

Just as group fasting can be beneficial, group mindfulness sessions can amplify the experience. Sharing a space with like-minded individuals, all striving for a deeper understanding and connection, can provide motivation, camaraderie, and a shared sense of purpose.

Incorporating mindfulness into fasting is not about complicating the process but enriching it. It's about transforming fasting from a mere act of abstention to a holistic journey of discovery, acceptance, and growth. As each individual delves deeper into this journey, they'll find that the blend of fasting and mindfulness offers a path to not just physical well-being, but emotional and spiritual harmony as well.

Celebrating Small Wins and Progress

In a world that often emphasizes the destination over the journey, it's easy to overlook the smaller achievements that pave the way to larger goals. Especially within the realm of fasting, where the emphasis often lies on tangible outcomes like weight loss or health metrics, recognizing and celebrating the tiny steps and milestones can profoundly impact one's psychological well-being and motivation.

1. The Psychology of Celebration:

The act of acknowledging and celebrating progress, no matter how small, releases dopamine, the neurotransmitter responsible for feelings of pleasure and reward. This release not only offers immediate gratification but reinforces the behavior that led to the success, thus creating a positive feedback loop that encourages consistency and persistence.

2. Defining Personal Wins:

What constitutes a 'win' is deeply personal. For some, it might be sticking to the fasting schedule for a day, while for others, it could be the realization of a deeper connection with their body's signals. Establishing these personalized benchmarks ensures that the journey remains tailored to the individual's unique experience and goals.

3. Daily Reflections:

Dedicating a few moments at the end of each day to reflect on the fasting experience can unearth numerous small wins. Perhaps it was the successful navigation of a social event without breaking the fast or the newfound ability to differentiate between emotional and physical hunger. Recognizing these moments daily magnifies their significance.

4. Visualization:

Visualization is a powerful tool where one imagines a desired outcome, instilling a deeper belief in its attainability. When paired with celebrating small wins, it acts as a reminder of both the journey traversed and the path ahead, fostering optimism and determination.

5. Sharing Wins:

Sharing one's achievements, regardless of their size, creates a ripple effect. It offers an opportunity for communal celebration, amplifying the joy and offering motivation to others on a similar journey. Whether through support groups, with loved ones, or on social platforms, shared celebrations create a sense of community and interconnectedness.

6. Non-Food Rewards:

Within the context of fasting, it's crucial to decouple the concept of rewards from food. Instead, think of rewards like a spa day, a new book, a walk in nature, or any other experience that offers joy and relaxation without centering around food.

7. Embracing the Non-Linearity of Progress:

Progress is rarely a straight line. There will be days of immense clarity and growth, followed by days that feel stagnant or even regressive. Celebrating small wins is a reminder that every step, regardless of its direction, offers valuable lessons and insights.

8. The Power of Affirmative Self-Talk:

The narratives one tells oneself play a crucial role in shaping experiences and beliefs. By framing each small win with positive affirmations and self-talk, one strengthens the foundation of self-belief and confidence. Statements like "I am capable", "Every step matters", or "I trust my journey" can serve as powerful anchors.

9. Documenting the Journey:

Maintaining a visual or written record of progress offers tangible evidence of the journey's evolution. It could be in the form of photographs, journal entries, or even voice notes. Over time, this compilation serves as a testament to the multitude of small wins and their collective significance.

10. Prioritizing Mental Well-being:

While fasting offers numerous physiological benefits, the psychological journey is equally vital. Celebrating small wins underscores the importance of mental well-being, reminding individuals that while the body is being nourished and healed through fasting, the mind requires equal care and attention.

11. Setting New Benchmarks:

With every small win celebrated, it's essential to set new benchmarks. This continuous cycle of setting, achieving, celebrating, and then resetting ensures that the journey remains dynamic, challenging, and rewarding.

12. The Role of Gratitude:

Gratitude and celebration are deeply intertwined. By cultivating a practice of gratitude, one shifts the focus from what is yet to be achieved to what has already been accomplished, however minute. This perspective not only amplifies the joy of small wins but offers a more holistic view of progress.

13. Recognizing Internal Changes:

Not all wins are visible. Some of the most profound changes during the fasting journey are internal, be it a shift in mindset, a deeper connection to one's body, or heightened emotional intelligence. Recognizing and celebrating these intangible wins is crucial, as they form the bedrock of lasting change.

14. Embracing Joy in the Present:

While it's natural to set goals and work towards them, it's equally vital to find joy in the present. Celebrating small wins is a reminder that happiness and contentment need not be deferred until a larger goal is achieved. They can be embraced and experienced in the here and now.

15. The Broader Impact:

The act of celebrating small wins during one's fasting journey transcends the individual experience. It serves as a beacon of hope and motivation for others, demonstrating that progress is multifaceted and that every step, irrespective of its size, holds value and significance.

In the grand tapestry of the fasting journey, it's the multitude of small wins that weave together to create a narrative of growth, resilience, and transformation. By recognizing, valuing, and celebrating these moments, one not only enhances their own experience but offers inspiration to countless others on similar paths. It's a testament to the power of the present moment and the myriad ways in which progress can manifest, reminding all that in the pursuit of larger goals, it's the journey that holds the true essence of transformation.

10

The Fasting-Fatigue Connection

Understanding Energy Production during Fasting

Energy, the force that keeps us moving, thinking, and thriving, is intricately produced by the body in various ways. It might seem counterintuitive to think that our bodies can maintain energy levels, let alone produce energy, during a fast when no external food source is consumed. Yet, our physiology has evolved in remarkable ways to keep us functioning even in the absence of immediate food intake. Let's delve into how this works, particularly during fasting.

Our body derives energy primarily from three macronutrients: carbohydrates, fats, and, to a lesser extent, proteins. In our everyday, fed state, our body typically relies on the energy from the carbohydrates we consume, breaking them down into glucose that our cells use as a primary energy source. This process involves the hormone insulin, which facilitates the transport of glucose into cells.

However, during fasting, glucose availability dwindles as we deplete the stores of glycogen (a form of stored carbohydrate) in our liver and muscles. With the body's preferred source of quick energy running low, a shift in metabolism takes place. The liver begins the process of gluconeogenesis, where it generates glucose from non-carbohydrate sources such as certain amino acids.

Simultaneously, our body taps into its vast reservoir of energy stored as fat. Fat cells release fatty acids, which are transported to the liver and converted into molecules called ketones, especially beta-hydroxybutyrate. This state is referred to as ketosis, and these ketone bodies effectively replace glucose as the primary source of energy for many cells, including crucially, the brain.

Contrary to some misconceptions, ketones are an efficient and potent energy source. Some even argue that the brain operates more effectively on ketones than on glucose. This shift is an evolutionary adaptation, ensuring that our ancestors could function, think clearly, and hunt or gather food even when food was scarce.

However, it's essential to note that the transition from glucose burning to fat burning isn't always seamless. As the body adjusts to this new energy source, some people might experience what's popularly referred to as the "keto flu," characterized by fatigue, headaches, and mood swings. This phase is temporary, and as the body becomes more adept at using fat for fuel, these symptoms generally subside.

Proteins, the third macronutrient, play a less direct role in energy production during fasting. The body generally avoids breaking down proteins for energy unless absolutely necessary, such as in prolonged starvation. This is because proteins are vital for other functions, like repair and enzymatic processes. Nonetheless, some amino acids can be converted into glucose through gluconeogenesis, as mentioned earlier, but this is not the body's primary or preferred method of energy production during a fast.

Furthermore, the role of hormones in energy regulation during fasting cannot be overlooked. Cortisol, a stress hormone, sees a rise, playing a part in mobilizing energy stores. Growth hormone levels also increase, which helps preserve muscle tissue and encourages the utilization of fat stores for energy.

Adiponectin, a hormone released from fat cells, increases during fasting and has been linked with increased fat oxidation and improved insulin sensitivity. Leptin, another hormone from fat cells, usually decreases during fasting. Leptin's primary role is signaling satiety or fullness to the brain. Its decrease might signal the brain about the scarcity of food, leading to adaptive behavioral and metabolic responses.

Interestingly, fasting also activates a process called autophagy. It's like the body's housekeeping service, cleaning out damaged cells and regenerating new ones. While autophagy doesn't directly produce energy, it plays a role in maintaining cellular health, ensuring cells function optimally and efficiently.

While it's fascinating to understand these mechanisms, it's equally essential to recognize that everyone's experience with fasting varies. Factors such as genetics, initial body composition, overall health, and even the microbiome can influence how one feels during a fast and how efficiently these energy production processes operate.

The body's ability to switch energy sources during fasting is a testament to its adaptability. It reminds us that fasting isn't about deprivation but rather about understanding and harnessing the body's innate capabilities. The next segments of this chapter will explore how to combat potential fatigue during fasting, ensure vitality, and delve into the relationship between sleep quality and fasting.

Combatting Fatigue and Ensuring Vitality

Fasting, for all its benefits, can bring about challenges. Fatigue is a frequently reported symptom, especially for those new to the fasting experience or undergoing longer fast durations. It's essential to address this aspect not only from a comfort standpoint but also to ensure the fasting journey is sustainable and beneficial in the long run.

Understanding the origins of fatigue during fasting can help in devising strategies to combat it. Fatigue can arise from various factors, ranging from the metabolic shifts in the body, dehydration, imbalances in electrolytes, to even psychological elements associated with the act of abstaining from food.

When the body transitions from using glucose to fats as its primary energy source, the aforementioned "keto flu" can kick in. While this state is temporary, the symptoms can be intense, with fatigue being a prominent feature. Ensuring that the body makes this transition smoothly can mitigate feelings of tiredness.

A well-structured fasting regimen will aid this process. For individuals new to fasting, it's advisable to start with shorter durations and gradually increase as the body adapts. This approach offers the body a chance to acclimatize to its new energy sources slowly.

Hydration plays a pivotal role in warding off fatigue. While fasting, especially in the absence of food which naturally contains water, the body can dehydrate faster than one realizes. Dehydration can rapidly lead to feelings of tiredness and sluggishness. Therefore, it's of utmost importance to drink adequate water throughout the fasting period. Some individuals find it beneficial to add a pinch of salt to their water to maintain electrolyte balance, which can also prevent feelings of fatigue.

On the topic of electrolytes, these are minerals that have an electric charge, crucial for various bodily functions, including nerve signaling, muscle contractions, and maintaining fluid balance. Common electrolytes include sodium, potassium, calcium, and magnesium. When fasting, especially during longer durations, there can be a significant loss of these electrolytes, leading to symptoms such as fatigue, headaches, and even muscle cramps.

Regularly consuming bone broths or electrolyte-infused drinks (without added sugars) can help replenish these minerals. It's also beneficial to be aware of the symptoms of electrolyte imbalance and take corrective measures promptly.

Physical activity, while fasting, is a topic of debate. Some argue for complete rest, while others vouch for the benefits of light to moderate exercise. There's no one-size-fits-all answer. However, engaging in some form of movement, like walking or gentle stretching, can increase circulation, improve mood, and alleviate feelings of fatigue. For those who are used to more intense workout regimens, it might be a good idea to adjust the intensity and duration during fasting days.

The psychological aspects of fasting can also contribute to feelings of fatigue. The very knowledge that one isn't consuming food can lead to a perceived sense of tiredness. Mindfulness practices, meditation, or engaging in activities that serve as a distraction can be beneficial. Remember, a significant portion of the fasting experience is mental. Retraining the mind to understand that the absence of food doesn't necessarily equate to immediate energy depletion can help combat feelings of fatigue.

Nutrient deficiencies can also play a role in inducing tiredness. Even outside of fasting periods, if one's diet lacks essential vitamins and minerals, fatigue can manifest. It's crucial to ensure that meals consumed during eating windows are nutrient-dense and balanced. A diet rich in leafy greens, lean proteins, healthy fats, and whole grains can provide the body with the necessary building blocks to function optimally. In some cases, supplements might be necessary to address specific deficiencies. However, it's always recommended to consult with a healthcare professional before incorporating any supplements.

Sleep is another dimension intertwined with fasting and fatigue. The quality and quantity of sleep can significantly influence energy levels during a fast. Interestingly, some people report improved sleep during fasting, while others might experience disturbances. It's essential to establish a healthy sleep routine, ensuring that one gets adequate and restful sleep, particularly during fasting periods.

Fasting is a deeply personal journey, with each individual's experience being unique. While the general guidelines mentioned above can help combat fatigue and ensure vitality, it's important to remember that everyone's body reacts differently. Listening to one's body, making adjustments when necessary, and seeking support, be it through communities or professionals, can make the fasting journey smoother and more beneficial.

Ensuring vitality during fasting isn't just about staving off fatigue. It's about optimizing the body's potential, harnessing the benefits of fasting, and creating an experience that nourishes both the body and the mind. As the chapters progress, the relationship between sleep quality and fasting will be explored further, shedding light on this intricate dance of rest and abstention.

Sleep Quality and Fasting: What's the Link?

Sleep, a fundamental human need, intertwines with every facet of health, including digestion, cognition, mood, and metabolic functions. It stands to reason that dietary patterns, including fasting, can have a profound impact on sleep quality. Delving into the science and experiences of many reveals a multifaceted relationship between fasting and sleep.

Beginning at a cellular level, the circadian rhythm, often termed the "body clock," regulates sleep-wake cycles. This rhythm not only determines sleep patterns but also plays a role in feeding times. Every cell in the body has its clock, all of which are coordinated by the master clock in the brain. There's a growing body of evidence suggesting that fasting and feeding can influence and be influenced by these clocks.

For instance, the onset of melatonin, a hormone responsible for sleep initiation, can be affected by food intake. Eating close to bedtime can delay melatonin secretion, potentially pushing the onset of sleep to later than desired. Fasting, which often involves abstaining from food during the evening hours, might benefit individuals by aligning food intake with the body's natural circadian rhythm, leading to improved sleep onset.

Conversely, the act of fasting can, in some individuals, stimulate alertness. The body's evolutionary response to food scarcity was to heighten alertness, aiding in food search. This heightened state, while beneficial during day-time fasts, can potentially disrupt sleep if fasting extends into the late evening.

Glucose metabolism is another piece of the puzzle. As previously discussed, fasting transitions the body from glucose to fat metabolism. This switch can have varying effects on sleep. Ketone bodies, produced during fat metabolism, have been shown to have a role in the sleep-wake cycle. Some individuals report deeper sleep and more vivid dreams during extended fasts, which could be attributed to increased ketone production.

However, a sudden transition into fasting, especially for those unaccustomed to it, can lead to disturbed sleep patterns. This disturbance could be due to a combination of factors, including changes in metabolism, hormonal fluctuations, and even the psychological aspect of knowing one is fasting.

Ghrelin, often termed the "hunger hormone," also has a role in sleep regulation. During fasting, especially in the initial stages, ghrelin levels can surge. While its primary role is in signaling hunger, ghrelin also has an influence on sleep architecture. Elevated ghrelin levels can affect the proportion of REM (Rapid Eye Movement) sleep, a critical phase of sleep responsible for dreams and memory consolidation.

Additionally, fasting has an influence on the stress hormone cortisol. While short-term fasting can elevate cortisol levels, potentially leading to sleep disturbances, longer-term, well-adapted fasting routines might stabilize cortisol rhythms. It's essential to be aware of this, especially for individuals who already have disrupted cortisol patterns, such as those with chronic stress or adrenal fatigue.

Electrolyte balance, as mentioned in the previous section, plays a role in muscle function and nerve signaling. Imbalances, especially during extended fasts, can lead to muscle cramps or restless legs, both of which can disturb sleep. Ensuring adequate intake of minerals such as magnesium can promote muscle relaxation and improve sleep quality.

Considering the complex interplay of these factors, what steps can one take to ensure optimal sleep during fasting?

Alignment with Circadian Rhythms: Aligning fasting windows with natural circadian rhythms, such as fasting during the evening and night and eating during daylight hours, can support natural sleep patterns.

Gradual Transition: For those new to fasting or shifting to more extended fasting durations, a gradual transition can prevent sudden disruptions in sleep.

Mindful of Meal Timing: The last meal before a fast should ideally be 2-3 hours before bedtime, ensuring that digestion doesn't interfere with the onset of sleep.

Electrolyte Balance: Consuming bone broths or supplements to ensure an adequate electrolyte balance can prevent sleep disturbances due to muscle cramps.

Stress Management: Engaging in relaxation techniques, be it meditation, deep breathing exercises, or gentle stretching, can lower cortisol levels and promote restful sleep.

Sleep Environment: This remains a cornerstone of good sleep hygiene. A dark, cool, quiet environment can significantly enhance sleep quality.

Remember, individual experiences with fasting and sleep can vary. What might aid one person's sleep could disrupt another's. It's a journey of discovery, requiring adjustments and fine-tuning to find the perfect balance.

Further ahead, the exploration of managing stress during fasting provides deeper insights into the cortisol connection and tools to balance this crucial hormone. Sleep, while a restful act, requires proactive measures during fasting to ensure its quality and restorative powers remain uncompromised.

Managing Stress to Optimize Fat Burning

Stress, an innate response sculpted by evolution, once served as a survival mechanism, preparing our ancestors to face immediate threats. However, in today's frenetic world, stressors have shifted from fleeting physical dangers to sustained emotional, psychological, and environmental challenges. This constant state of heightened alertness and the hormonal cascades it induces can significantly impact metabolic functions, including fat metabolism.

Cortisol, commonly referred to as the "stress hormone," plays a central role in this narrative. Under acute stress, cortisol's immediate surge acts beneficially, mobilizing energy reserves and sharpening mental acuity. This mechanism was essential for survival situations, but when these acute stress responses turn chronic, the persistently elevated cortisol can wreak havoc on various physiological systems, especially fat metabolism.

Chronic stress and consistently high cortisol levels can lead to a slew

of metabolic disturbances:

Insulin Resistance: Cortisol increases the release of glucose into the bloodstream to prepare for the "fight or flight" response. In situations of chronic stress, this continuous glucose surge can desensitize insulin receptors, leading to insulin resistance, a precursor to weight gain, especially around the midsection.

Appetite Dysregulation: Elevated cortisol can increase appetite and cravings for high-calorie, sugary, and fatty foods. Such foods provide a temporary surge in serotonin, a feel-good neurotransmitter, explaining the appeal of "comfort foods" during stressful times.

Decreased Fat Oxidation: High cortisol levels can reduce the body's ability to burn fat for energy, favoring glucose utilization instead. This can be particularly counterproductive during fasting, where the primary goal is to shift to fat metabolism.

Muscle Catabolism: Chronic stress can lead to muscle breakdown, a process where the body taps into amino acids for immediate energy. This reduction in muscle mass can drop the basal metabolic rate, further compounding fat gain.

Digestive Disturbances: Stress can impair gut function, leading to issues like bloating, inflammation, and altered gut microbiota. Such disturbances can further hinder optimal nutrient absorption and metabolism.

In the realm of fasting, managing stress becomes paramount, not just for psychological well-being, but to maximize the potential fat-burning benefits. Here are strategies to keep stress in check:

Mindfulness and Meditation: The power of mindfulness, the practice of staying present, can significantly reduce perceived stress. Meditation, a structured form of mindfulness, has shown to reduce cortisol levels, enhancing the mental and physiological response to stress.

Deep Breathing Techniques: Deep, diaphragmatic breathing can activate the parasympathetic nervous system, offering a counter-response to the stress-induced sympathetic activation. Breathing exercises can serve as immediate relief during moments of heightened stress.

Exercise: Physical activity, be it brisk walking, yoga, or more intensive workouts, can act as a potent stress-reliever. Exercise stimulates the release of endorphins, natural painkillers that can elevate mood.

Nature Immersion: Spending time in nature, often termed "forest bathing," can lower cortisol levels, reduce blood pressure, and improve mood. Even brief periods in natural settings can confer significant stress-relief benefits.

Limit Stimulants: Caffeine and certain medications can increase cortisol production. While some coffee during fasting can boost fat metabolism, excessive intake, especially in stress-prone individuals, can be counterproductive.

Prioritize Sleep: As explored in the previous section, quality sleep is crucial for stress management. A rested mind and body can better cope with daily stressors, preventing chronic cortisol elevation.

Connect Socially: Positive social interactions can release oxytocin, a hormone that can counteract cortisol. While fasting might introduce some social restrictions, maintaining social connections remains crucial.

Seek Professional Support: Persistent stress, especially when interfering with daily functioning or causing significant distress, warrants professional intervention. Therapists or counselors can offer tailored coping strategies.

Maintain a Balanced Fasting Approach: It's essential to remember that fasting, especially when rigorous, can introduce a form of physiological stress. Balancing fasting duration and intensity, as tailored to individual needs, ensures that the practice remains beneficial rather than an added stressor.

Engage in Pleasurable Activities: Hobbies, listening to music, reading, or engaging in any enjoyable activity can act as a stress buffer, creating moments of relaxation and contentment.

Understanding the intricate relationship between stress and fat metabolism offers a broader perspective on the holistic nature of well-being. Fat loss, often viewed through the narrow lens of diet and exercise, gains depth when framed within the larger context of mental and emotional health.

The subsequent section explores the potential role of supplements during fasting, offering insights into how certain compounds can support both physiological and psychological aspects of the fasting journey. Remember, the interplay of body and mind remains integral to the overarching narrative of health, and managing stress stands as a pillar in this holistic endeavor.

Supplements to Consider During Your Fasting Journey

While the essence of fasting revolves around abstaining from food for specific durations, the body's requirements for certain nutrients don't disappear. Especially when engaging in prolonged fasts, certain micronutrients can deplete faster than others, potentially causing imbalances. This section delves deep into the world of supplements that might bolster a woman's fasting journey, ensuring vitality, hormonal balance, and the prevention of deficiencies.

The complex synergy of fasting and female metabolism necessitates particular attention. Thus, when considering supplements, it's crucial to understand that it's not about replacing food but about ensuring optimal health.

Electrolytes: When fasting, especially during extended periods, the body tends to excrete more electrolytes than usual, especially if fluid intake increases. Essential electrolytes include sodium, potassium, magnesium, and calcium. These are crucial for muscle function, nerve function, and maintaining fluid balance. A good electrolyte supplement can make all the difference in preventing symptoms like cramps, dizziness, or even heart palpitations.

Vitamin D: Renowned for its role in bone health, immune function, and mood regulation, Vitamin D is often deficient in many women, regardless of whether they fast. When fasting, the limited food intake can further reduce the intake of this crucial vitamin. It's also notable that Vitamin D has a role in insulin sensitivity, a key aspect of fasting benefits.

B Vitamins: These are a group of vitamins essential for energy production, brain function, and the synthesis of hormones. While many B vitamins are stored in the body, they are water-soluble, and consistent intake is necessary for optimal health. Especially B12, commonly found in animal products, can be a concern for women who practice plant-based fasting.

Iron: This is especially important for menstruating women. Iron is essential for the production of red blood cells and for transporting oxygen in the blood. A deficiency can result in fatigue, dizziness, and reduced immune function. However, it's crucial not to overdose, so always get tested before supplementing.

Omega-3 Fatty Acids: Renowned for their anti-inflammatory properties and essential for brain health, Omega-3 fatty acids can support a woman's fasting journey. They can help with mood regulation, hormone synthesis, and cell function. Opt for a high-quality fish oil or algae-based supplement for vegetarians and vegans.

Adaptogens: While not essential nutrients, adaptogens like Ashwagandha, Rhodiola, and Holy Basil can support the body's stress response. They can potentially help with the cortisol spikes some women experience during fasting, ensuring a balanced mental and physical response to the fasting challenge.

Zinc: Another mineral that plays a role in immune function, wound healing, and hormone synthesis. It's especially important for thyroid health. Again, a balanced intake is crucial as excessive zinc can interfere with copper absorption.

Probiotics: Intermittent fasting can have profound effects on gut health. While abstaining from food, the gut gets a 'break', which can help with the balance of good bacteria. A good probiotic can assist in maintaining this balance, supporting digestion, and overall gut health.

Coffee and Green Tea Extracts: Not essential, but these natural stimulants can provide an energy boost during fasting windows. They also contain antioxidants and can support fat burning. However, they're to be used with caution, especially in women sensitive to caffeine or those who experience anxiety.

While this list is by no means exhaustive, it highlights the main supplements that can potentially support a woman during her fasting journey. It's essential to remember that everyone's body is different. It's always best to consult with a healthcare professional before starting any supplement regime, especially when fasting. Testing and understanding one's unique requirements can make the fasting journey more tailored, effective, and health-promoting.

As we wrap up this chapter, remember that fasting is a tool – a way to reconnect with oneself, to heal, to discover, and to grow. Supplements are there to support this journey, to ensure it's undertaken with the utmost respect for the body's intricate needs.

The next chapter, 'The Future of Feminine Fasting', looks towards what's on the horizon, diving into the prospects and possibilities that lie ahead for every woman embarking on this transformative journey.

11

The Future of Feminine Fasting

Personalizing Fasting: Future Advancements

The realm of fasting has been an evolving landscape, deeply intertwined with human evolution, religious practices, and modern health movements. As we've navigated through the nuances of feminine fasting, we've discerned that a one-size-fits-all approach is far from ideal. With the marriage of science and technology, the future of fasting is brimming with possibilities tailored to individual needs, genetic predispositions, and specific health outcomes. Personalized fasting stands as a beacon in this futuristic landscape, heralding an era where the fasting protocol becomes as unique as one's fingerprint.

Genomics and Fasting: Our genes are a treasure trove of information. Every individual carries genetic markers that influence metabolism, hormone production, and response to food deprivation. As genomics advances, we find the capability to decode these markers, offering bespoke fasting plans. Imagine knowing that your genetic makeup leans towards shorter fasts or requires specific nutrient replenishment post-fast. These insights will revolutionize fasting paradigms.

Wearable Technology: Wearable tech has already made its mark in tracking steps, heart rate, and sleep patterns. The next frontier is real-time tracking of metabolism-related indicators. Devices will soon be able to monitor ketone levels, blood glucose, and even hormone fluctuations. With this data at one's fingertips, adjusting fasting windows, intensity, and nutrient intake becomes a precise science.

Microbiome Mapping: The gut's microbial landscape is an orchestra, playing a symphony that affects digestion, immunity, and even mood. Personalized fasting will harness knowledge from one's microbiome. If certain beneficial bacteria thrive better in longer fasting windows or if specific foods post-fast foster a balanced gut, this information can reshape fasting protocols.

Hormonal Health: Fasting impacts hormonal health, and each woman's hormonal profile varies. As medical science progresses, at-home hormone testing kits will become mainstream. These kits, combined with AI-driven platforms, will provide insights into how fasting should be tailored around one's menstrual cycle, menopause status, or even conditions like PCOS.

Virtual Nutritional Coaches: Artificial Intelligence will play a pivotal role in guiding individuals through their fasting journey. Imagine a virtual coach, armed with all your health data, providing real-time advice. Feel a sudden energy dip? Your virtual coach will advise on whether to break the fast or how to support your body through it.

Fasting Retreats and Spas: The concept of wellness retreats is not new. However, the future will see establishments dedicated solely to personalized fasting. These retreats, equipped with medical professionals, nutritionists, and wellness experts, will design fasting regimens based on in-depth health assessments. An individual will experience fasting as a holistic journey, complete with meditation, targeted physical activities, and nutrient-rich meals.

Personalized Fasting Foods: With the food industry continually innovating, there will be a surge in products tailored for those on specific fasting regimens. Think of foods designed to replenish exact nutrients post-fast, based on individual requirements. These might be fortified with specific minerals, vitamins, or even beneficial bacteria, ensuring that breaking a fast becomes an optimized process.

Emotional and Mental Health Integration: Fasting is not just a physical endeavor. It's an emotional and mental journey. Future advancements will include platforms and tools that integrate emotional health. Mood tracking, guided meditation sessions tailored to fasting phases, or even virtual reality experiences that support mental clarity during fasting will emerge.

Community Building Platforms: The sense of community amplifies the fasting experience. Advanced platforms will emerge, connecting individuals based on their fasting protocols, challenges, or goals. These will be spaces for shared experiences, knowledge exchange, and mutual encouragement.

Research and Data: As more women embark on their fasting journeys, there will be a surge in data. This data, when analyzed, will provide deep insights, refining fasting protocols and enhancing benefits. We're at the cusp of understanding fasting's profound effects on conditions like endometriosis, fibroids, or even postpartum recovery. The data will lead the way.

In this brave new world of personalized feminine fasting, empowerment is the key. The ability to understand one's body at a micro-level and make informed decisions will redefine the fasting narrative. It will no longer be about enduring challenges but about embarking on a harmonious, science-backed journey. This blend of technology, science, and self-awareness promises a future where fasting becomes a joyful, transformative experience, intimately woven into the fabric of a woman's life.

Fasting During Different Life Stages: Pre-Menopause, Menopause, and Beyond

Every woman's journey is punctuated by various life stages, each with its unique metabolic, hormonal, and physiological nuances. As time's tapestry unfurls, the female body undergoes profound shifts, from the vibrant rhythms of youth to the serene wisdom of older age. Fasting, as a health and spiritual tool, must adapt and evolve in tandem with these stages. As we project into the future, understanding and customizing fasting for each stage becomes paramount.

Pre-Menopause: This phase, often spanning a woman's late 30s to early 50s, is marked by subtle shifts. Hormone levels start to fluctuate, and women may experience changes in menstrual cycle regularity, intensity, or even mood swings.

Hormonal Synergy: Estrogen and progesterone start their gradual descent during this phase. Balancing these hormones becomes crucial. Personalized fasting during this stage might involve shorter fasts during the luteal phase when progesterone is dominant, ensuring mood stability and energy balance.

Metabolic Adjustments: As metabolism may begin to slow down, fat accumulation can become a concern. Intermittent fasting, especially the 16:8 or 14:10 protocols, can aid in maintaining metabolic rate and preventing unwanted weight gain.

Bone Health: Ensuring bone density becomes essential. Fasts during this phase can be complemented with weight-bearing exercises and post-fast meals rich in calcium and Vitamin D.

Menopause: Often perceived as a challenging stage, menopause is a natural transition. As menstrual cycles cease, estrogen levels significantly drop, ushering in a new physiological state.

Hot Flashes and Fasting: Hot flashes, a common symptom, can be influenced by blood sugar levels. Personalized fasting in the future may use real-time blood sugar monitoring to adjust fasting windows, mitigating intense hot flashes.

Mood and Mental Clarity: Declining estrogen can influence neurotransmitters like serotonin. Fasting protocols during menopause might incorporate specific break-fast meals that are rich in tryptophan, a precursor to serotonin, ensuring mood balance.

Bone and Heart Health: Post-menopause, the risk of osteoporosis and heart diseases increases. Future fasting guidelines may recommend shorter but more frequent fasts, combined with post-fast meals that are rich in omega-3 fatty acids, magnesium, and calcium.

Beyond Menopause: As women journey into their 60s and beyond, health priorities shift. The focus leans heavily towards longevity, vitality, and cognitive health.

Cognitive Health: One of the promising areas of fasting research is its impact on brain health. Fasting activates autophagy, a cellular cleanup process, and boosts brain-derived neurotrophic factor (BDNF). Personalized fasting for senior women might involve regular short fasts, ensuring neural pathways remain vibrant.

Muscle Preservation: Sarcopenia, or muscle loss with age, becomes a concern. Combining protein-rich post-fast meals with resistance training can become a standardized recommendation.

Digestive Health: As digestion slows down with age, fasting can offer the digestive system much-needed breaks. Personalized fasting might involve gentler fasting-mimicking diets, ensuring digestive wellness.

Longevity and DNA Repair: Fasting influences sirtuins, proteins linked with longevity. As we gather more data on genetic markers linked with longevity, fasting can be tailored to activate these markers, promoting a longer, healthier life.

Each life stage offers its challenges but also its unique beauty. Embracing these stages with a tailored fasting protocol ensures that women don't just navigate these transitions but thrive. The blend of ancestral wisdom and cutting-edge science offers a holistic roadmap, honoring the female body's rhythms and cycles. This roadmap not only promises health and vitality but also deepens a woman's connection with herself, making each life stage a celebration of feminine essence.

Fasting in the Modern World: A Tool for Lifelong Health

In the undulating tides of human history, every epoch has its unique challenges. The modern world, with its bustling cities, digital landscapes, and relentless pace, presents a set of challenges previously unfathomed. Amidst the cacophony of notifications and the allure of convenience foods, the ancient practice of fasting emerges, not as a relic of bygone days, but as a potent tool for lifelong health.

Urban Living and Detoxification: Modern cities, while hubs of innovation, are also epicenters of pollution. Air, water, and even our foods carry toxins. Fasting acts as a reset button, activating the body's innate detoxification processes. Liver, kidneys, and even the skin get a break from constant exposure, enhancing their capacity to cleanse and rejuvenate.

Digital Overload and Mental Clarity: The modern mind is inundated with information. The constant barrage can lead to mental fog and reduced cognitive capacity. Fasting, by reducing the energy expended on digestion, redirects this energy towards brain function. This makes fasting a potent tool for those in professions demanding high cognitive function.

Convenience Foods and Metabolic Health: Processed foods, high in sugars and unhealthy fats, are omnipresent. The modern diet can lead to metabolic imbalances, insulin resistance, and obesity. Fasting, by offering intervals where insulin levels drop, can restore metabolic health. In the future, as more becomes known about the harmful effects of certain food additives, fasting might be prescribed specifically to counteract these effects.

Stress and Hormonal Balance: The relentless pace of modern life puts the body in a perpetual state of fight or flight. Chronic stress can disrupt hormonal balance, especially cortisol levels. Fasting helps recalibrate the body's stress response, ensuring hormonal harmony.

Modern Ailments and Cellular Health: Diseases like type 2 diabetes, cardiovascular ailments, and even certain cancers are termed 'lifestyle diseases' because they're heavily influenced by modern living patterns. Fasting, especially when combined with a healthy lifestyle, acts at a cellular level. Processes like autophagy, where cells self-cleanse, are activated during fasting, offering protection against these ailments.

Sleep Quality in the 24/7 World: With round-the-clock entertainment, work pressures, and artificial lighting, quality sleep is compromised. Fasting, by regulating circadian rhythms and hormonal patterns, can improve sleep quality. Future homes might come with smart devices that track fasting windows and adjust room lighting accordingly, promoting sync with natural circadian rhythms.

Social Connectivity and Community Fasts: While the digital age connects us globally, there's an increasing sense of isolation. Community fasts can emerge as platforms for real, tangible connections. Virtual platforms can transform into physical community centers, where group fasts are observed, combined with activities like meditation, yoga, or group discussions.

Sedentary Lifestyles and Energy Management: With automation and technology, physical activity has taken a backseat. Fasting can counteract some of the negative effects of a sedentary lifestyle. By enhancing mitochondrial function, fasting ensures that cells produce energy efficiently, even with reduced physical activity.

Sustainability and Conscious Consumption: The modern world is waking up to the perils of overconsumption. Fasting, at its core, is about conscious deprivation. As more people adopt fasting, there's a collective shift towards valuing resources, be it food or even time. This can have far-reaching effects on sustainable living and conscious consumption patterns.

Personal Growth and Spiritual Quests: Personal development and spiritual quests are gaining momentum in the modern age. Fasting, with its roots in spiritual traditions, can become a sought-after tool for those looking for inner growth. Retreats offering fasting as a means to delve deep within might become more prevalent.

In a world where external stimuli are in overdrive, fasting offers an inward journey. It's a voyage of self-discovery, of understanding one's body and mind. As the challenges of the modern world escalate, so does the potential of fasting to counteract them. Women, armed with the knowledge and tools to harness fasting's power, can navigate the modern maze with grace, vitality, and resilience. The modern world, with all its complexities, becomes not a labyrinth but a playground where the empowered woman dances to her rhythm, with fasting as her steadfast ally.

Community Fasting: Building Support and Shared Experiences

At the crossroads of individual intention and collective endeavor lies the phenomenon of community fasting. Historically, shared rituals of abstaining from food have been deeply rooted in various cultures, spanning across religions, geographies, and eras. Today, as the health benefits of fasting take center stage, the concept of community fasting emerges with renewed vigor, transitioning from a predominantly religious ritual to a wellspring of mutual support, camaraderie, and shared human experience.

The Power of Shared Intent: When individuals come together with a shared goal, the collective energy can amplify individual resolve. Fasting, with its myriad of physical, emotional, and even spiritual challenges, can sometimes become a daunting journey when trodden alone. In a community setting, the combined intentions serve as a scaffold, lending strength, motivation, and the drive to persevere.

Emotional Support during Challenges: No two fasting journeys are identical. Each woman may face unique challenges, be it physical discomfort, emotional upheavals, or moments of self-doubt. A community setting provides a platform where experiences are shared, advice is sought, and comfort is found. Simply knowing that others are experiencing similar challenges can provide solace and strength.

Collective Knowledge and Insights: As fasting gains traction in medical and wellness circles, new research, findings, and insights are continually emerging. Community fasting platforms can become hubs of knowledge sharing. From understanding the nuances of female metabolism, tailoring fasts to menstrual cycles, to sharing recipes that nourish post-fasts, the collective wisdom of a community often surpasses individual knowledge.

Social Engagement and Bonding: Fasting can sometimes lead to feelings of isolation, especially in cultures or families where regular meals are central to social interactions. Community fasting events, whether they're weekly meet-ups, monthly potlucks, or annual retreats, provide opportunities for social engagement. Bonds forged during these gatherings often transcend the act of fasting, leading to deep, lasting friendships.

Accountability and Motivation: Knowing that others are invested in one's fasting journey can be a powerful motivator. Regular check-ins, shared milestones, and even gentle nudges during moments of temptation can make the difference between giving up and pressing on. Community members often hold each other accountable, ensuring that the path, though challenging, is never abandoned.

Shared Rituals and Celebrations: Humans, by nature, are ritualistic beings. Shared rituals, be it breaking a fast together, celebrating milestones, or even simple practices like group meditations during fasting windows, can infuse the journey with a sense of purpose and joy. These rituals often become anchors, grounding individuals during the tumultuous tides of fasting.

Diverse Perspectives and Inclusivity: A community is often a melting pot of diverse backgrounds, cultures, and experiences. This diversity can offer a rich tapestry of perspectives on fasting. From cultural nuances, traditional practices, to modern adaptations, the myriad viewpoints can offer a holistic understanding of fasting, making the practice more inclusive and adaptable.

Online Platforms and Digital Communities: The digital age has shrunk the world, making it possible for individuals from far-flung corners of the globe to come together. Online community fasting platforms, forums, and even mobile applications can offer support, knowledge, and camaraderie without geographical constraints. These digital platforms often serve as the first touchpoint, leading to physical meet-ups and deeper connections.

Community-led Research and Advocacy: As the benefits of fasting become increasingly evident, there's a growing need for more research, especially focused on female physiology. Communities can play a pivotal role in advocating for research, pooling resources, and even volunteering for studies. Such grassroots movements can propel fasting to the forefront of wellness and medical interventions.

Evolving Traditions and Creating New Ones: As community fasting becomes more prevalent, there's a possibility of evolving age-old traditions, adapting them to contemporary needs, and even forging entirely new rituals. These might become part and parcel of societal norms, passed down generations, making fasting an integral part of human evolution.

In essence, community fasting intertwines individual aspirations with collective endeavors. It reminds women that while their fasting journey is deeply personal, they're never alone. There's a tribe, a sisterhood, standing with them, cheering them on, sharing their challenges, and reveling in their triumphs. This shared experience not only amplifies the benefits of fasting but also elevates it to a celebration of collective human spirit, resilience, and unity.

Closing thoughts: Your unique fasting journey and the path ahead

The echoes of women throughout history have left footprints that indicate the power and resilience inherent in the female spirit. One such testament to this enduring strength is fasting, a practice that has been passed down through generations, not as a mere ritual but as a tool of liberation, empowerment, and rejuvenation. Today, as we stand on the cusp of an era that embraces holistic health and individualized wellness, the future of feminine fasting becomes even more significant.

It's undeniable that fasting is no longer just about abstaining from food. It is an art and science, and as women, it's essential to recognize and understand the interplay of hormones, metabolism, psychology, and physiology. The synchronization of all these elements makes each woman's fasting journey a unique masterpiece. This chapter aims to provide a forward-looking perspective, one that serves as a beacon to the uncharted territories of female fasting.

Personalizing fasting: Future advancements

With advances in technology, it's foreseeable that personalizing fasting will become the norm. Imagine a wearable device that not only tracks your heart rate, sleep patterns, or steps but also monitors hormonal fluctuations. Such devices could provide real-time feedback, allowing women to adjust their fasting durations and intensities according to their unique physiological needs.

Genetic testing might soon play a pivotal role in determining fasting protocols, offering insights into how one's genes affect fasting tolerance, fat storage, and even hunger pangs. In a world where data reigns supreme, embracing these innovations can transform the fasting experience, ensuring it's not just effective but also safe and sustainable.

Fasting during different life stages: Pre-menopause, menopause, and beyond

Throughout a woman's life, she undergoes several significant hormonal shifts. The beauty of fasting lies in its adaptability. During pre-menopause, for instance, women might find they benefit from shorter, more frequent fasting intervals. As one transitions into menopause, hormone replacement therapy or other treatments could affect fasting needs. The post-menopausal years, with their unique set of challenges, could be navigated with adjusted fasting protocols, focusing more on maintenance and metabolic health. The mantra remains the same: listen to your body and adapt.

Fasting in the modern world: A tool for lifelong health

Urbanization and the modern-day lifestyle often stand at odds with healthful living. Increased stress levels, exposure to pollutants, erratic sleep schedules, and the ubiquity of processed foods make maintaining optimal health a challenge. Fasting emerges as a beacon, a tool that offers respite from the incessant onslaught of modern-day stressors. By regularly practicing fasting, women can not only manage their weight but also fortify themselves against chronic diseases, boost cognitive health, and foster emotional well-being.

Community fasting: Building support and shared experiences

The rise of digital platforms and social media has made it easier than ever to build and find communities. Virtual fasting groups offer spaces for women to share their experiences, challenges, and successes. These platforms are not just about motivation; they are about education, shared learning, and creating a tapestry of collective experiences. Women, by nature, thrive in collaborative environments, and this sense of community can be the catalyst that drives adherence to fasting and maximizes its benefits.

The path ahead is not just one of individual journeys but a collective movement. A movement where every woman, armed with knowledge, empowered by community support, and inspired by personal successes, moves forward in her unique fasting journey.

Every chapter of "Her Fast, Her Freedom" has aimed to shed light on the multifaceted nature of fasting for women. It is a journey, one filled with discovery, challenge, empowerment, and transformation. As you embark or continue on your fasting odyssey, remember that this is not about fitting into a mold or adhering to a one-size-fits-all approach. It's about carving out your path, one that respects your body's cues, celebrates its uniqueness, and propels you toward holistic well-being.

Your fast is your freedom, and your future awaits. As you stride ahead, know that you are not alone. In this ever-evolving world of feminine fasting, you are a pioneer, a beacon, and a testament to the timeless strength of women. So, embrace the future, for it is bright, and it is yours.